Introduction
to Oral Preventive Medicine

A program for the first clinical experience

Hans R. Mühlemann

Translated from the German by
Thomas M. Hassell, D.D.S., Dr. med. dent., Department of Pathology,
in collaboration with
Alfred L. Ogilvie, D.D.S., M.S., Department of Periodontics,
University of Washington, Seattle, U.S.A.

Buch- und Zeitschriften-Verlag "Die Quintessenz" 1976
Berlin, Chicago, Rio de Janeiro and Tokyo

Title of the German edition: "Einführung in die orale Präventivmedizin"
Copyright Hans Huber Publishers, Berne/Switzerland

Copyright © 1976 by Buch- und Zeitschriften-Verlag "Die Quintessenz",
Berlin, Chicago, Rio de Janeiro and Tokyo

Type setting and printing: Kupijai & Prochnow, Berlin
Binding: Lüderitz & Bauer, Berlin

ISBN 3 87652 591 8

Table of Contents

Introduction to the English-Language Edition

The reader of this English-language version of Professor Hans R. Mühlemann's *Einführung in die orale Präventiv-Medizin* may find the following comments helpful.

The original German-language book presents a series of 16 exercises introducing beginning dental students to virtually all aspects of dentistry. Despite the wide ranging content of the course, all dental teachers, regardless of their particular interests, have welcomed it, because it provides students a solid base upon which they can build. The purpose is to augment, not to supercede, existing programs.

This English edition has been revised and to a certain extent expanded, because it is intended for use not only as a workbook of "programmed instruction" for dental students but also as a "refresher course" for practicing dentists. The theoretical portions introducing each chapter have been reworked in such a way that the practitioner can reap significant intellectual and practical benefit even if it is not possible for him to participate in an actual course. The Results Sheets included at the end of each chapter show the reader what results he might have obtained if he *had* performed the practical exercises.

The exercises described herein were first performed at the Dental Institute, University of Zurich, Switzerland, under the direct supervision of Professor Mühlemann and his staff. The book was developed over several years, as experience and student feedback showed the way to a final presentation.

Our goal in preparing this English edition has not been to merely translate German words into English, but rather to put Professor Mühlemann's *ideas* into English. Because Mühlemann is an intense, dynamic person with a quick mind, his thoughts often seem to range far ahead of his words; he talks in a staccato style, seemingly to make up for the time lag. His German-language original is written in much this way, and rightly so, since it was intended for use by his own students and staff. But because we hope that the English edition will be used the world over by those who know of Mühlemann's work but don't know him personally, we felt that a somewhat less frenetic style would be more appropriate.

We were tempted at first to delete Professor Mühlemann's rather frequent references to continental Europe and to things Swiss in particular. In the end, we incorporated the Swiss "flavor," deciding it was indeed suitable for an international audience.

Perhaps the greatest challenge was transposition of Mühlemann's illustrative limericks into adequate English, a task not always successfully completed. We rejected some suggestions that the limericks be deleted altogether; Mühlemann without dry humor is not really Mühlemann at all. In short:

> Translating Mühlemann is fun.
> He's witty — a master of pun.
> His limericks sensational
> Are so educational.
> Forget about classroom hum-drum!

Professor Mühlemann did not review this manuscript before it went to press. We like to think he would have approved it if he had.

Thomas M. Hassell
Alfred L. Ogilvie

Seattle, August 1975

What is the purpose of this course?

This book was prepared primarily for the instructor. Many young teachers today are convinced of the necessity for a broader presentation of preventive medicine. But oftentimes an instructor will procrastinate, because he is aware of the time involved in organizing such a program. This book should be welcomed by these teachers, because it gives them the wherewithall on the one hand to present a course without a tremendous investment of time, and on the other hand represents a collection of material which has proven beneficial for both dental students and dental hygiene students.

The central focus of this course is not gray theory, but rather observation of living things, of persons. Results gathered by students during the course may be compared to data in the literature. In this way, the often tiresome statistical reports in textbooks and journals suddenly become meaningful. Automatically, the question-and-answer game will begin; for example: Why is it that in Swedish studies the severity of gingival inflammation in students is considerably different from Swiss? What factors could be responsible for this difference? This book lays down the biological bases of prevention. The student comes to know the purpose of prevention and is motivated to practice it.

Introduction

Dental medicine today finds itself in a pervasive state of change. Numerous generations of dentists, while they stood at the treatment chair with their drills in their hands, were concerned with nothing else except how to repair carious lesions. Why did they never become more curious? Each decade brought new technological advances for easing or eliminating drudgery and busywork: the whining air turbine replaced the foot-driven handpiece; pharmacological progress made possible painless treatment; the age of plastics gave us new materials and simplified therapy. Dental technique has approached perfection and has achieved something that no other medical specialty has been able to do: dentistry has put to use each new technological development quickly and effectively. It is not surprising that young people are attracted to this type of perfection, to this fight for the highest precision.

That is one side of the coin. Should the other side be forbidden the hopeful student? Despite all the technical perfection, many an older dentist is dissatisfied with his life's work, seeing it merely as a constant process of tooth repair. He has experienced for himself the disappointment of seeing the primary dentition lost due to caries, only to be replaced by a permanent dentition which, apparently according to some unwritten law, is filled, then filled again, then crowned, then extracted. He participates in tooth replacement, first by bridgework, then by partial dentures and finally by a set of complete dentures. Why can't the situation be different? Many a father of a large family has fearfully asked himself this question, if only for purely financial reasons. Official spokesmen of the dental profession admit openly that "reparative dentistry" cannot provide adequate treatment for all levels of society. Yet "adequate," as they use the term, need not mean "expensive." A healthy oral cavity does not have to be full of gold. Nobody knows this better than dentists themselves. Thousands of them chew for years on temporary fillings, which seemingly are never replaced by definitive restorations because of a crowded waiting room and the lack of time.

The solution of the "dental problem" requires a *new orientation of dentistry*. The basis for this must be the recognition and acceptance of the fact that, in the long run, the *prevention of dental diseases is just as important, practically speaking, as is therapy of same.*

In Switzerland, the dentist-to-population ratio is such that about 2,200 persons must be cared for by each dentist. Dental treatment in terms of care for dental *and* periodontal destruction would require at least twice as many practitioners. In view of the impossibility of achieving a dentist-to-population ratio of 1,000:1, one has no choice but to *reduce the incidence of disease by one-half.* This represents the social medicine aspect of the "dental problem."

Does a dentist who practices "preventive dentistry" achieve self-satisfaction with his profession? One cannot contest that the treatment of a carious defect, i. e., artful preparation and filling of a cavity, represents craftsmanship and an art form which gives tremendous satisfaction. One has set out upon a task, proceeds self-critically with the necessary manipulations, and stands before the result of one's perfectly performed work of art. But over the course of time, the failures return, although many of them remain undetected or are chalked up to the patient's lack of proper oral hygiene or to "soft teeth" which the unfortunate patient inherited from his parents . . .

A preventive measure, the topical application of fluoride for example, will only be performed by a practitioner who has been convinced of its efficacy and who believes in it. This is a difficult thing for every student to grasp: he paints a fluoride solution onto a tooth and waits, in vain, for a visible reaction… Treatment and result, fluoride application and caries-freedom, lie years apart. However, the happiness and professional satisfaction will come with time to the patient dentist. He will be able to observe, for example, that the numerous children of a large family, treated conscienciously with preventive measures, will require very few fillings, and that their mouths will remain almost completely caries-free.

"Preventive dentistry" does not mean only the *prevention of a disease*, it also implies the *early detection and the timely and simple treatment* of the clinical manifestations of the disease.

The early stages of periodontal disease, and this applies in some degree to dental caries as well, are often *reversible*. The diagnosis of initial symptoms motivates especially toward prevention. Microsymptoms require precise examination and observation. The patient himself can diagnose a hole in his tooth, but the early detection of a carious lesion, or the first infammatory alterations in the periodontium and the oral mucosa is a more difficult thing. Precise observation implies the collection of quantitative data. The preventive-minded practitioner is not satisfied with merely knowing whether or not a patient has gingivitis. He wants to know the *extent* and the *intensity* of the pathological alterations, because these are prerequisites for the prevention of further damage or for the reversal of already existing disease. Prevention is a scientific process. Therefore, it does not exist without quantitative findings ("data").

One purpose of this book is to spare the student, during his first contact with dentistry, from the shock which the author's generation had to experience: tray after tray filled with thousands of formaldehyde-soaked extracted human teeth. The first command I can remember was: "Come in! Throw out those with no caries! (How ironic!) Drill 'em! Fill 'em!" The natural science and biological studies I had pursued before entering dental school appeared to be merely luxurious ballast.

In our opinion, the very first clinical experiences in dentistry should be based upon knowledge and experience which the new dental student has already achieved from a broad theoretical course of university-level studies. This is very meaningful where the field of prevention is concerned. *Introduction to Oral Preventive Medicine* is built upon this concept and has as its purpose the motivation of the clinical beginner towards quantitative observations and a critical view of both the literature and his instructors in the clinic. It seems to us that this course offers a means for educating dentists and modern dental auxiliaries who are motivated toward prevention.

Introduction to Oral Preventive Medicine was written for a learning *team:* student instructor and dentist learn from each other and with each other. The team should find both learning and the performance of the practical exercises easier with this program. This is the reason for the "cook book" style of the text.

Nothing would make this author happier than to find this book hopelessly outdated 10 years from now. It would mean that real progress had occurred. This course of work and study would then have been worthwhile indeed.

H. R. Mühlemann

Leitmotiv for Oral Preventive Medicine

1. The basis for preventive medicine is scientific fact. Only with this basis can we achieve real progress in the form of better health and less disease.

2. The arch enemy of true progress is dogma. Dogma blinds and manipulates. Beware of the teacher who tells you, "it is so."

3. Allow yourself to be convinced only by scientific facts. You are studying at a university, which, through you, should serve the public. Only the best is good enough for the public.

4. Cherish the teacher who admits that his assertions are open to discussion.

5. No one can forbid you to believe. Wherever scientific facts are lacking, belief is the alternative. But belief, like religion, must be declared.

The Scientific Facts

I. In the dogmatic lecture hall

Lecturing professor:

"The minute you discover even the tiniest carious lesion on a tooth, it must be filled immediately. Otherwise, the dental pulp will be diseased in a few months."

Pseudostudent (writing down every word without looking up):

"Interesting"!

Student untrained in stenography, probably a thinker:

"I haven't been to the dentist for 4 years. At that time, the dentist told me I had to have a beginning carious lesion filled as soon as possible. I've observed it since then. It hasn't gotten any bigger."

Professor (glaring):

"You observed incorrectly! How could you, an absolutely inexperienced beginning student, understand anything at all about dental caries? Your observation is unfounded and contradicts my vast experience in thousands of cases. It is so"!

Suicide candidate (student):

"Where can I review your thousands of cases"?

Professor (Dr. med., Dr. med. dent., Dr. h. c. sci., Ph. D., F.A.C.D. etc.):

"My modesty does not permit me to publish all my studies." (He clears his throat) "I would not be standing here if I were not telling the truth."

II. In the scientific lecture hall

Teacher (without necktie):

"Although one hears it again and again, it is not true that the initial carious lesion progresses to pulpal disease in a few months."

Modern student:

"On what do you base this claim"?

Teacher (considered an "upstart" by his academic colleagues, because he wears no necktie):

"I'm happy that you accept only scientific facts and not mere claims or opinions. I have brought along a published investigation which supports my statements."

Disgruntled student (with necktie):

"A great deal of material gets published; some believe too much. Paper is patient."

Teacher:

"Yes, but this publication is by an internationally renowned author; his name is Marthaler."

Critical student:

"That expression you just used is impressive. But just how do you measure this quality called 'international renown'"?

Teacher:

"Once you get into the literature, especially the Anglo-Saxon literature, you will soon discover that the 5 or 10 best-known oral epidemiologists in the world cite Marthaler's work again and again in their publications. In other words, Marthaler's publications are recognized as the scientific blocks with which other scientists build. If you want still more evidence, try looking through the "Science Citation Index"[1]. Judge for yourself the value of this Index as a measure of the competence of any scientist.

[1] Request literature about the Science Citation Index from:
Institute for Scientific Information, 325 Chestnut Street, Philadelphia, Pa. U.S.A. 19106

Orientation article:
Margolis, J.: Citation indexing and evaluation of scientific papers. Science 155:1213, 1967.

In principle, in the S.C.I. one finds how often a scientific publication from any given author is cited elsewhere. It has been demonstrated that valuable, creative publications are more often cited than pseudoscientific articles."

Numerous students:

"But we can't read English."

Teacher:

"That is most unfortunate. The language of biological and medical science today is English. I'm tempted to compare you with aspiring mountain climbers who have no ropes."

Female student:

"Are you going to abandon us without a 'rope'"?

Teacher (big-hearted):

"I really mean it. I would suggest that you skip several of my courses in order to make time to study English. You would benefit much more, because you have an entire life in front of you. Without a working knowledge of English, you'll be in no position to start out in any profession based on science. You will always regret your failure to master English."

Impatient student:

"Where was this study by Marthaler published"?

Teacher (an editor in his spare time):

"In Helvetica Odontologica Acta, Volume 16, page 69, 1972."

Student (dumbfounded):

"A Swiss journal in the English language? Treason"!

Teacher (apparently well-documented):

"Yes, sir. In the language of science. By this means, a journal reaches 3 to 4 times as many of those who are truly interested. Wouldn't it be a bad investment for the Swiss to publish research data, which has required hundreds of hours to accumulate and analyze, in a form which would be read by only a few people"?

Student (impatient):

"That may be, but it is still no guarantee that this particular publication by Marthaler has high scientific quality or makes valid statements about the rate of progression of carious lesions."

Teacher (addicted, lighting a cigarette):

"You are perhaps not aware that the leading journals in the field of dentistry, such as the Journal of Dental Research, Archives of Oral Biology, Caries Research, the Journal of Periodontal Research, Acta Odontologica Scandinavica and Helvetica Odontologica Acta do not publish any article until it has been submitted to a panel of experts for critical analysis. Suggestions for improvement are made by these referees, so that vague points will be clarified, thus making the article more valuable. Marthaler has probably never published a manuscript which has not first been reviewed by experts in the field. Only the lay press can't wait."

Student (coughing, a passive smoker): "Let's get to the point."

Teacher (more considerate):

"Marthaler examined 133 seven to fourteen-year-old children in the city of Zurich for carious lesions and the growth of same over a 7-year period."

Student (well prepared):

"How did he do the examining? I've read that even just the lighting conditions can influence the results of an examination."

Teacher (knows Marthaler):

"Dr. Marthaler knows that, too. He also knows the percentage of error in his examination technique. He knows as well the main factors responsible for the variations in his data. In reality, his study group is only a random sample. It is for this reason that there are also confidence limits associated with his mean values. On the basis of these, it is possible to make statements about a population with a certain mathematical probability that the random sample is representative of the population as a whole."

Insistent student:

"From Marthaler's study one sees that an initial proximal-surface carious lesion, as detected on the radiograph, requires an *average* of 25 months to progress from the most superficial enamel layer to the inner half of the enamel. But as future dentists, an average value doesn't help us very much. We'll be taking care of individual people."

Teacher (fortunately not only a clinician but also a person with some experience in epidemiology):

"Marthaler provides not only average values, but also the distribution, the mean variation and the range of the individual values. In this example the mean was 18 months. Of the total of 283 lesions studied, 141 had progressed into the inner half of the enamel in less than 18 months, while 141 required more than 18 months for the same degree of progression. In the total of 283 initial lesions studied, Marthaler found only 23 which had invaded the inner half of the enamel layer within 6 months. 49 lesions required more than three years, several up to five years to penetrate the same distance."

Student:

"So, in any given individual case, one still doesn't know how rapidly an initial lesion will progress."

Teacher (fortunately not just a theoretician, but also with a great deal of clinical experience):

"If you look at the initial lesion by itself, yes. But if you observe the condition of the entire oral cavity – the dentition, its over-all caries prevalence, the localization and distribution of the carious lesions, the patient's oral hygiene and the condition of the gingivae – then you will be able to decide, even in the individual situation, whether the probability of galloping rampant caries is high or low. Furthermore, you will be able to decide whether to place a filling immediately, or to wait and see.

But we will deal with these considerations a bit later. For the moment we must realize simply that, thanks to the results of an investigation performed using scientific methods, thanks to scientific facts, we are in a position to make correct judgements in a practical situation. These judgements are not based upon assumptions or theories or dogma or upon 'thousands of observations not published because of modesty.'

By the way, are you aware that we have only discussed the permanent teeth and not the primary teeth?"

You may read more about caries progression in these articles:

Backer-Dirks. O.: Posteruptive changes in dental enamel. J. Dent. Res. 45, 503; 1966.

Van Erp, N.A.K.M. and Meyer-Jansen, A.C.: A caries study of the temporary molars and its significance for their regular conservative care. Netherlands Dent. J. Supp. 5, 77, 51; 1970

Rugg-Gunn A.J.: Approximal carious lesions. A comparsion of the radiological and clinical appearances. Brit. Dent. J. 133, 481; 1972.

Berman, D.S. and Slack, G.L.: Caries progression and activity in approximal tooth surfaces. a longitudinal study. Brit. Dent. J. 134, 51; 1973.

A recent article by Marthaler, T.M. and Wiesner, V.: Rapidity of penetration of radiolucent areas through mesial enamel of first permanent molars. Helv. Odont. Acta 17, 19–26; 1973.

Conclusion

Do not allow yourself to be manipulated by dogmatic claims.

Recognize only the authority of the scientific facts.

Beware when everything appears simple and logical.

Dogmatic teachers are good salesmen.

Organization of the Course

The *active participation of the student in the various exercises* is the axis around which the course revolves. Because the student enters as an absolute beginner where observation of the oral cavity is concerned, the first portion of each exercise must deal with theory.

Before proceeding to the practical exercises, I will devote a few pages to a brief overview of dental caries, the periodontal diseases and the etiologies of these oral pathological conditions.

The quality of a course always depends upon the quality of its organization. The student, in his early helplessness, appreciates a step-wise, systematic progression. Teachers who in the future may want to organize similar courses can easily adapt this outline to fit their own special wishes and circumstances. Also, several chapters may be combined if that is desired.

An unconventional method of presentation often makes it necessary to adopt a rather staccato literary style, in order to avoid long-windedness. Some readers may criticize the course sequence, but one must not forget that it is precisely the sequence of a course which plays such an important role in motivation for thinking. Pure memorization of knowledge is *not* the most important thing.

The ideal time requirement for this course is 16 weeks of 5 to 6 hours per week. The number of participants should not be less than 20, because otherwise it will be impossible to make valid comparisons of the students' results with those in the literature.

Experience has shown that the optimal student-to-instructor ratio is 4-to-1. A 6:1 ratio is the maximum.

The theoretical portion presupposes elementary knowledge of oral structural biology. As mentioned before, the first encounter is with a broad consideration of the two disorders most often observed in the oral cavity. With this background, we will then proceed to the exercises, which deal with more specific aspects of oral pathology and its prevention.

Brief Overview of Dental Caries and Periodontal Disease

Dental caries and periodontal disease are by far the most common diseases affecting the oral cavity. Both of these disorders are chronic, tissue-destructive processes. The major portion of a practicing dentist's professional life is devoted to the treatment of dental caries and periodontal disease, and to consequences and complications arising from them.

Dental Caries

Definition

Dental caries is a decalcifying and decomposing process in enamel and in dentin which begins at a predilection site on the tooth surface and then invades the deeper structures of the tooth.

Dental caries is a disease of civilization. *Caries* is the term for the disease entity; the morbid process itself, along with its characteristic symptoms is the *carious lesion.*

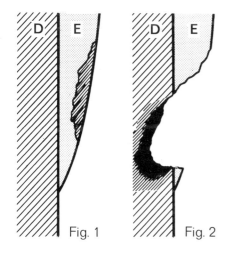

Fig. 1   Fig. 2

D = dentin
E = enamel

The *initial lesion*
(enamel lesion, Fig. 1)

The initial lesion consists of a partial decalcification of the dental enamel with maintenance of the enamel structure. It is easily observed on a dried tooth as an opaque chalky spot. It is also called "enamel caries."

The *advanced lesion*
(dentin lesion, Fig. 2)

The advanced lesion exhibits the transition from partial to total decalcification of the enamel. The destructive process expands into the dentin by means of demineralization and tissue decomposition, and becomes an obvious defect, a "hole" in the tooth called "dentin caries."

The *predilection sites* of carious lesions are determined by the morphology of the tooth crown and the relative positions of the teeth. Essentially, these are areas where microbial deposits (plaque) can grow undisturbed.

Clinically, a distinction is made between:

Fissure lesions

("occlusal caries", Fig. 3)

Pit lesions (Fig. 3)

These are found primarily on the palatal aspect of maxillary molars, the buccal surface of mandibular molars and on the lingual surface of upper incisors.

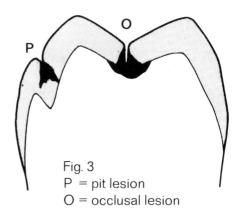

Fig. 3
P = pit lesion
O = occlusal lesion

Smooth surface lesions (Fig. 4)

These appear most often as cervical enamel lesions (chalky spots).

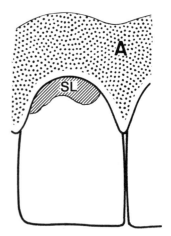

Fig. 4
A = attached gingiva
SL = smooth surface lesion

The untreated carious lesion almost always leads with time to inflammatory pulpal infection (pulpitis).

Proximal surface lesions (Fig. 5)

These are localized near the proximal contact area between the teeth. The initial mesial or distal enamel lesion is difficult to diagnose clinically. Radiographic diagnosis is more predictable.

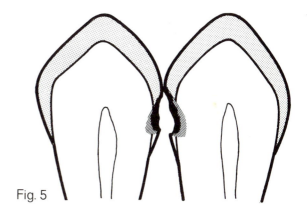

Fig. 5

Cementum caries (Fig. 6)

This results from carious destruction of root surfaces exposed at the cervical region.

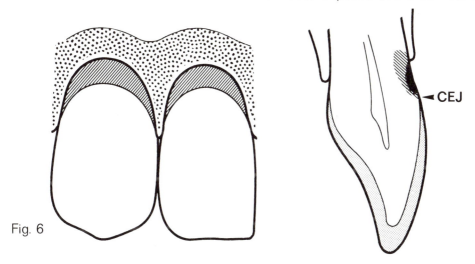

Fig. 6

◄CEJ

Secondary caries (Fig. 7a–b)

Secondary caries is the term used to describe carious lesions which develop at the margin of a previously placed restoration.

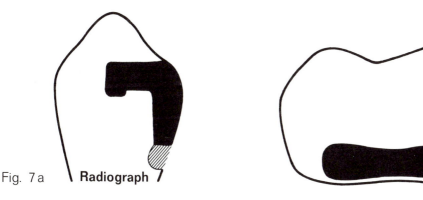

Fig. 7a   **Radiograph**   Fig. 7b

Etiology of Dental Caries

The primary causes of caries are exclusively of external, local nature.

1. Dental plaque (microbial deposits)

The dental plaque is really a bacterial colonization which is firmly adherent to a hard surface, such as a tooth or a prosthesis. Everything that promotes plaque accumulation is *potentially* cariogenic: for example, oral uncleanliness, tooth positional anomalies; improper fillings and poorly contoured crowns present so-called retention zones. The slogan "No bacteria, No caries!" emphasizes the importance of mechanical and chemotherapeutic measures for oral hygiene in caries prevention.

2. Fermentable carbohydrates

If dental plaque is exposed to a fermentable substance, for example a sugar solution, lactic acid is formed immediately due to enzymatic glycolysis. The resting pH of plaque falls within a few minutes from approximately 6.7, to 4.0 (the so-called Stephan curve, see Fig. 14). At the "critical pH" of ~5.5, enamel is decalcified.

All mono- and disaccharides are rapidly fermented to acids. Only sucrose plays an additional role in plaque genesis. Certain plaque Streptococci can synthesize from sucrose the sticky extracellular polysaccharides (levans, dextrans, mutans) which cement plaque bacteria together. This promotes the accumulation of microbial deposits on the teeth.

"No fermentable carbohydrates, no caries!" This slogan also points out the significance of a rationally regulated intake of sugar, both for caries prevention and, as we shall see, for the prevention of gingivitis as well.

There are two additional oral factors which can determine the incidence of dental caries to a great degree:

a. An abundant flow of saliva

The bicarbonate buffer system of stimulated saliva can partially neutralize the acids produced by plaque. This clarifies the role of the hard, saliva-stimulating foodstuffs in caries prevention! On the other hand, a dry mouth (xerostomia) promotes caries and gingivitis.

b. A high fluoride content of the enamel surface

High fluoride content inhibits enamel demineralization by acids produced in the plaque. This is one of several ways in which fluoride aids in the prevention of dental caries.

24

Caries in art:

> Dentists in the Louvre supposed
> That Mona Lisa's lips are closed
> To hide her deep cavities
> And other oral depravities
> Which Da Vinci, no doubt, opposed.

Literature

König, K.G.: Karies und Kariesprophylaxe. Goldmann Pocket Book (Taschenbuch) Me 17, 1971.

Periodontal Disease

Definitions

Periodontium: Tissues which support the tooth root when the tooth crown is subjected to mechanical force loading. Includes the periodontal ligament, radicular cementum, part of the alveolar bone and the marginal gingiva.

Periodontal disease: Destructive process beginning at the gingival margin and progressing chronically through the periodontium, leading to a gradual loosening of the tooth and its eventual loss.

Types of lesions

1. Noninflammatory periodontal disease (periodontal atrophy)

Due to *recession* of the marginal gingiva *and* the crest of the alveolar bone, the tooth neck and the coronal portion of the tooth root become exposed. Simultaneously the attached gingiva (A) becomes narrower and narrower. Clinically, this process can proceed even in the absence of inflammation (Fig. 8a, b).

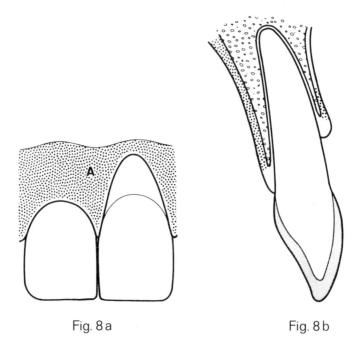

Fig. 8 a   Fig. 8 b

2. Inflammatory periodontal disease (marginal periodontitis)

Inflammatory periodontal disease always begins with an inflammation of the marginal gingiva which surrounds the neck of the tooth like a collar. This inflammation is termed *gingivitis* (Fig. 9), or, if only the col region is involved, *papillitis.*

a. Gingivitis

Gingivitis is not periodontitis, but there is no periodontitis without gingivitis.

Cause

The cause of gingivitis is dental plaque in immediate contact with the papilla (interdental space) or with the marginal gingiva. Systemic factors, e.g., pregnancy or diabetes mellitus, can intensify the degree of gingival susceptibility to inflammation, but by themselves can never cause gingivitis.

Symptoms

The earliest symptom of gingivitis is bleeding from the gingival sulcus in the papillary or marginal regions upon careful probing (Fig. 10). Other (later) symptoms include discoloration (reddening, cyanosis) and swelling of the papilla or of the marginal gingiva, as well as increased flow of exudate (crevicular fluid) from the gingival sulcus.

b. Marginal periodontitis

Definition

The term marginal periodontitis should be used only when chronic gingivitis has led to actual destruction of the marginal periodontium. Characteristic events in this process include dissolution of the gingivodental and transseptal collagen fibers and of the marginal periodontal ligament, resorption of the marginal alveolar bone with subsequent epithelial proliferation, pocket formation and increased crevicular fluid flow ("pyorrhea alveolaris," Fig. 11).

The marginal destructive process can cause two types of *periodontal pockets:*

a. *Supraalveolar pockets or gingival pockets* (Fig. 12)

These consist of a deepening of the physiological gingival sulcus as a result of dissolution of the *supraalveolar* connective tissue and through resorptive *horizontal resorption* of the marginal periodontal bony structure.

b. *Infraalveolar pockets or bony pockets* (Fig. 13)

These are usually supraalveolar pockets in the early stages. Soon, however, vertical tissue destruction begins as well; the periodontal ligament and inner cortical bone of the alveoli are resorbed "perpendicularly" in the direction of the apex.

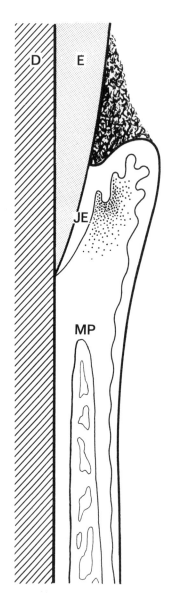

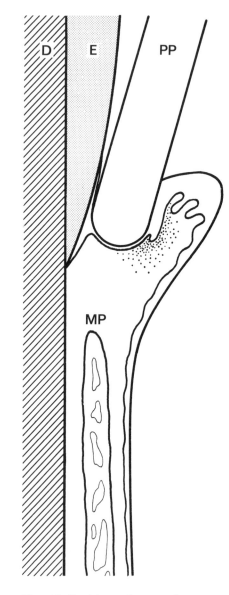

Fig. 9 Gingivitis

Fig. 10 Probing of normal gingival sulcus

D   = Dentin
E   = Enamel
JE = Junctional epithelium
MP = Marginal periodontal bone
PP = Periodontal probe
PE = Proliferating epithelium
R   = Resorption of bone

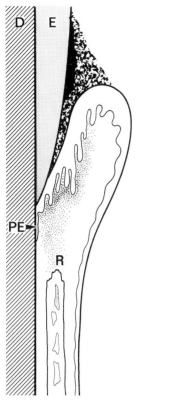

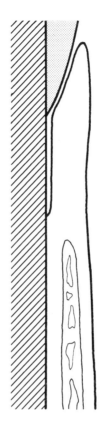

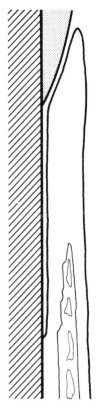

Fig. 11 Marginal periodontitis with beginning supraalveolar pocket

Fig. 12 Supraalveolar pocket

Fig. 13 Infraalveolar pocket

Pseudopockets arise due to swelling of the gingiva where the epithelial attachment is normal.

Periodontal disease in art:

> Mona's lips appear ill at ease,
> 'Cause Da Vinci'd concealed her disease.
> Microbial plaque in her sulci
> Created non-flattering ulci.
> Pyorrhea had caused her malaise!

Etiology of Marginal Periodontitis

Gingivitis, which represents the initial stage of the periodontal lesion, begins at the marginal and papillary gingivae, where the free gingiva is in immediate contact with the bacterial plaque. With time, the inflamed gingival tissues begin to break down, to be dissolved, and supraalveolar pocket formation is initiated.

The progression of the lesion into the deeper tissue components may be enhanced by periodontal trauma as well as by the dental plaque. This leads to periodontal disintegration, with infraalveolar pocket formation.

Everything which predisposes to plaque accumulation also leads to gingivitis, intensifies the severity of the lesion, and leads in time to periodontitis: poor oral hygiene, frequent intake of sugar, predilection sites resulting from anomalies of tooth position or poorly contoured dental restorations.

As is the case with gingivitis, systemic factors which increase susceptibiltiy to inflammatory stimuli can also accelerate the course of periodontitis.

An especially severe, but fortunately infrequently observed type of periodontitis has been termed *juvenile periodontitis,* when observed in children, or *periodontosis* when it occurs in adolescents or young adults. In these cases, deep infraalveolar bony pockets are created, which are believed to be the result of degenerative tissue alterations with superimposed inflammatory complications.

An international panel of renowned periodontologists attended a WORLD WORKSHOP IN PERIODONTICS* in 1966 in the United States. Because this learned panel refuted the very existence of "periodontosis," ("There is insufficient evidence to identify periodontosis as a specific disease entity"), "periodontosis" represents the nightmare of every clinical periodontist.

> R.I.P.:
>
> The Chairman announced with great glee:
> "Of periodontosis, at last we are free"!
> Like the ostrich with head in the sand
> The panel, with one sweeping command,
> Killed a lesion with *rhetoric,* see?

The precursor of periodontitis – gingivitis – begins in 80% of children almost immediately after the teeth erupt into the oral cavity. In 20-year-olds, periodontal pockets are a common finding.

---

* Proceedings published by S.P. Ramfjord, D.A. Kerr and M.M. Ash, Ann Arbor, Michigan, U.S.A.

Dental Plaque

The plaque may be compared to a living tissue: It consists of cells and intercellular substance (levans, mutans etc.). It grows and has a characteristic structure. New bacterial cells are produced, old ones die and are disposed of at the plaque surface, or are digested. The plaque has a characteristic metabolism.

Only a few minutes after a tooth has been thoroughly cleaned with a rotating brush and an abrasive paste, salivary mucoproteins from the oral fluid again begin to adhere to the enamel surface. During the next several hours, this layer of denatured mucin, known as the exogenous enamel covering or *pellicle*, begins to be contaminated by cocci and rod-shaped microorganisms from the oral fluid. If no oral hygiene is performed for the next 2 to 4 days, bacteria adherent to the pellicle will colonize. Discrete colonies form first, which later fuse to form a layer of microorganisms called *dental plaque*. During the early phase of plaque development, the most prominent microorganisms are aerobes or facultative anaerobes, such as:

facultative gram-positive Streptococci
aerobic gram-negative Neisseria (cocci)
aerobic gram-positive Leptotrichia (large filaments)
aerobic gram-positive Nocardia (small filaments).

As the plaque becomes thicker, *anaerobic* microorganisms begin to appear in the plaque microflora, among them:

Veillonella — gram-negative, very small cocci. Degrade lactic acid.
Actinomyces — gram-positive filaments
Corynebacteria — filaments
Fusobacteria — gram-negative rods and filaments.

On about day 10 of plaque growth, the obligate anaerobes such as Spirilla and Spirochetes begin to make their appearances. At about this time the plaque is completely formed; depending upon its localization, certain variations in the microorganism composition may be observed.

Plaque Metabolism

The metabolic processes of plaque are very complex. Fermentation, alkalinization, synthesis of carbohydrate polymers and the elaboration of inflammation-producing (phlogogenic) substances are functions which have been extensively researched. These will be described.

1. Plaque acidification due to fermentation or glycolysis[1]

Plaque may become acidic when fermentable substrate in the food we eat is metabolized by *acidogenic bacteria* within the dental plaque. Lactic acid produced in this manner causes enamel demineralization and carious lesions. The decrease in pH is known as the "Stephan Curve" (Fig. 14).

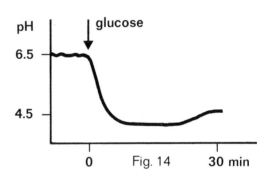

Fig. 14

2. Plaque alkalinization by ammonia production[1]

Some microorganisms have the ability to metabolize urea from the crevicular fluid and from the oral fluid, and this results in alkalinization of the dental plaque. Ureases within bacterial plaque split urea into ammonia and carbonic acid (Fig. 15). Alkalinity creates more ideal conditions for plaque mineralization, i.e., the formation of dental calculus.

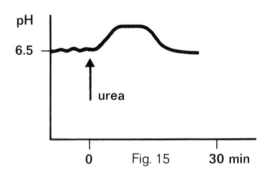

Fig. 15

Conversation overheard in dental plaque:

Veillonella whispered: "Methinks
That Nocardia with passion at me winks!
I love her because she's so sour,
But I must pine away every hour;
'Cause she takes only sugar-free drinks"!

---

[1] Kleinberg, I.: Regulation of the acid-base metabolism of the dento-gingival plaque and its relation to dental caries and periodontal disease. Int. Dent. J. 20, 451; 1670.

3. Synthesis of polysaccharides (polymers)[2,3]

Certain microorganisms polymerize sucrose to *extra*cellular glucans (dextran, mutan) and fructans (levans). Many microbes metabolize sucrose and other mono- and disaccharides to *intra*cellular glucans. Intracellular polymers serve as energy reserves for plaque bacteria. Extracellular polymers form the cementing substance which binds plaque to the tooth surface and which binds the bacteria within plaque to one another. The extracellular polymers also have roles to play in determining the permeability or semipermeability of dental plaque; in addition, they may serve as carbohydrate reserves, thus aiding in acid production.

Research with mutans[3]:

> A courageous Streptócoccal strain
> Attacked sugar molecules with disdain.
> Broke the chemical bond
> In this way was found
> Dr. Guggenheim's 1-3 mutane[4].

4. Phlogogenic substances

Plaque allowed to accumulate upon a perfectly cleaned tooth surface, in immediate contact with a healthy gingival margin, can cause inflammatory alterations after only a few days.

The inflammation is the result of this marginal, chronic *infection*. It does not occur as result of bacterial invasion. The plaque produces substances which loosen the cementing substance of the cells of the junctional epithelium (bacterial *enzymes* such as glucuronidase and hyaluronidase). Because of this increased permeability, high molecular weight plaque substances (e.g., *antigens*, endotoxins from bacterial membrane lipopolysaccharides) can also migrate through the epithelial attachment. Chemotactic substances, stemming either directly from the plaque or produced secondarily in subepithelial connective tissue (complement activation!), attract inflammatory cells to the site. These cells have in their lysosomes numerous tissue-digesting substances which can weaken the marginal connective tissue apparatus, and lead eventually to irreversible damage. In the realm of cellular immune reaction, substances are perhaps released which play a toxic role.

If the plaque is removed, the gingiva returns to normal in a few days. The greater the marginal accumulation of plaque, the longer and more intense is the marginal inflammatory reaction. Gingivitis permitted to persist for years usually progresses to marginal *periodontitis*.

[2] Gibbons, R.J., Socransky, S.S.: Intracellular polysaccharide storage by organisms in dental plaques. Arch. Oral Biol. 7, 73; 1962.

[3] Guggenheim, B.: Extracellular polysaccharides and microbial plaque. Int. Dent. J. 20, 657; 1970.

[4] Actually mut*an*, but the translator claims poetic license in this case!

Dental Calculus

Under certain conditions the dental plaque may become calcified. A prerequisite for mineralization is a slightly alkaline environment in the plaque. The calcification begins in small foci, which later become confluent. The process proceeds both within and between the plaque bacteria. Several minerals, principally brushite ($CaHPO_4 \cdot 2H_2O$), apatite $[[Ca_3(PO_4)_2]Ca(OH)_2]$ and whitlockite $[Ca_3(PO_4)_2]$ are formed. The surface of dental calculus is always covered with living, unmineralized, irritating plaque.

Supragingival calculus

Supragingival calculus is formed superior to the gingival margin. It has a tendency to form on tooth surfaces whose immediate vicinity is relatively alkaline, for example, the lingual aspect of mandibular incisors near the excretory ducts of the submandibular salivary gland, or the buccal surfaces of maxillary molars which are in proximity to the parotid gland ducts. Dental calculus forms not only on enamel, but also on foreign bodies such as restorative materials and prosthetic appliances.

Recently formed supragingivicial calculus is yellowish and relatively soft. As it ages, supragingival calculus often exhibits brownish discoloration and becomes harder.

Subgingival calculus

Subgingival dental calculus is formed in the region of the gingival sulcus, frequently accompanying marginal gingivitis. A prerequisite for formation of subgingival calculus is cervical plaque, which grows into the sulcus and mineralizes there. Subgingival calculus is often found in combination with supragingival calculus. Especially in the case of children, however, it may have no supragingival accompaniment other than plaque. It is dark brown in color and may be visible as a bluish discoloration through the marginal gingiva. It is very hard and adheres to the tooth more tenaciously than does supragingival calculus.

In cases of gingival recession, calculus which was originally formed subgingivally may be present as supragingival calculus.

Instructions for Use of This Teaching Manual

The first few pages of this book have presented a brief, theoretical introduction. We have made a rather critical consideration of the dogmatic and scientific aspects of the subject called preventive dental medicine, and we have had a short review of the nature of dental caries and periodontal disease. We also looked briefly at the etiologies of these two very important oral diseases. This material has lain the foundation for the subsequent course exercises.

The first page of each chapter presents an outline of the Exercise, including necessary materials. The subsequent Instruction Sheets present theoretical and introductory material which will provide the reader with information basic to an understanding of the meaning of each exercise. Then come the Exercise and Data Sheets, which describe the practical performance of exercises, and which often include predrawn charts for recording observations made. In a formal course, these Exercise and Data Sheets will be handed in to the instructor upon completion, for statistical analysis. Finally, the Results Sheets present the reader with the results of exercises performed by actual students at the University of Zurich Dental Institute from 1970 through 1973. In addition, comparisons are drawn with comparable data from the literature. I know of no other way to render "dry" oral epidemiological data so relevant and clear.

The exercise should always be demonstrated first, either in the lecture hall using visual aids, with a patient in the clinic, or in the laboratory. Subsequently, students choose partners. These pairs remain together throughout the course, each partner examining the other, or helping the other during the exercises. One student becomes the subject while the other is the examiner, and vice versa. In some cases, groups of three work out better. Here the third member records the data found by the second as he examines the first! It is extraordinary that in dentistry there are still some psychological hang-ups which appear when male and female students are asked to form pairs and examine each other. The situation, expressed in limerick form, is something like this:

"A mouth is a mouth," said the Prof.
"Pair up! At a partner don't scoff.
   Mixing these classes
   May require nitrous gasses,
Student hang-ups to banish, first off"!

Student Meier, when told to pair up,
Chose a shapely young thing (a D-cup!).
   But he just didn't dare
   To palpate and stare
In her mouth as at him she looked up!

The Clinical Treatment Area

Instruction sheets

I-1 a: Basic terminology in tooth numbering
I-1 b: Positioning the patient in the treatment chair
I-2 : Lighting

Exercise sheets

I-1 : The clinical treatment area

Material

Student: Responsible for bringing his own *clinic kit* (consists of mouth mirror, explorer, cotton pliers).

Instructor: Responsible for arranging dental unit lights, additional Miralux lamp, fiber-optic apparatus, tongue blades, protractor. Prepare unit for treatment of reclining patient.

Program

1. General introduction to course exercises
2. Discussion of the exercise with reference to Instruction Sheets
3. Division of the class into 4 groups for demonstrations. Rotation of the groups every 15 minutes. Subsequently, clinic exercises in groups of 2 or 3 students.

Group
Number   Demonstration

1   How to use the dental unit. Conventional (seated) position of the patient. Position of the dentist.
2   The operating light. Direct and indirect lighting using the mouth mirror. How to hold the mirror.
3   The unit light. Miralux lamp. Fiberoptic. Transillumination (Diaphanoscopy).
4   Sit-down dentistry with a reclining patient.

Basic Terminology in Tooth Numbering

Throughout this book, we will use the recently introduced "F. D. I." (Fédération Dentaire Internationale) system for tooth numbering. However, it must be recognized that several other tooth numbering systems have had wider use over the years. We will explain first the F.D.I. system, then the so-called International System, then the European System (which is still used to a great extent in Switzerland) and finally the Chevron System.

I. The F. D. I. tooth numbering system

This system was introduced in the early 1970's and was subsequently accepted by the Fédération Dentaire Internationale. It was developed to make possible the computerization of dental research data. It had been cumbersome or impossible to enter data into computers using tooth numbering systems common before 1970.
In the F. D. I. system, the four dental quadrants are numbered as follows:

Maxillary right = 1   Mandibular left   = 3
Maxillary left   = 2   Mandibular right = 4

Each quadrant has, potentially, eight teeth, and these are numbered from 1 through 8, beginning with the central incisor and moving posteriorly. Thus, the maxillary right central incisor is tooth number "1" in quadrant number "1". This tooth is designated verbally as "one, one," and written "11." Do not refer to this tooth as "number eleven," because - as we will see shortly - this will lead to confusion with a different numbering system. The figure below illustrates the F. D. I. system quite well.

Permanent teeth

Upper right								Upper left							
18	17	16	15	14	13	12	11	21	22	23	24	25	26	27	28
49	47	46	45	44	43	42	41	31	32	33	34	35	36	37	38
Lower right								Lower left							

Primary teeth

Upper right					Upper left				
55	54	53	52	51	61	62	63	64	65
85	84	83	82	81	71	72	73	74	75
Lower right					Lower left				

II. The international tooth numbering system

This is the system which is still used to a large extent in the United States today. It is a sequential numbering system. The maxillary right third molar tooth is called "number one." See the diagram below.

		A	B	C	D	E		F	G	H	I	J		
1	2	3	4	5	6	7	8	9	10	11	12	13	14	15	16

R ——————————————————————————————————— L

| 32 | 31 | 30 | 29 | 28 | 27 | 26 | 25 | 24 | 23 | 22 | 21 | 20 | 19 | 18 | 17 |
| | | | T | S | R | Q | P | O | N | M | L | K | | | |

Letters = primary teeth   Numbers = permanent teeth

III. The European tooth numbering system

In this system, the maxilla is the "plus" dental arch and the mandible is the "minus" dental arch. See the diagram below. The teeth of each quadrant are numbered from one through eight, beginning with the central incisor, thus the upper right cuspid is "three plus," and the lower left first molar is "minus six."

R   L

8+	7+	6+	5+	4+	3+	2+	1+	+1	+2	+3	+4	+5	+6	+7	+8
8–	7–	6-	5–	4–	3–	2–	1–	–1	–2	–3	–4	–5	–6	–7	–8

Primary teeth: 01, 02 etc., or I, II etc.

IV. The chevron system

This numbering system becomes clear upon inspection of the figure below.

	8		7		6		5		4		3		2		1			1		2		3		4		5		6		7		8

R ——————————————————————————————————— L

| 8| | 7| | 6| | 5| | 4| | 3| | 2| | 1| | |1 | |2 | |3 | |4 | |5 | |6 | |7 | |8 |

Before we can talk coherently about the oral cavity, there are several geographic terms with which we must become familiar. Refer to Figure I-1 below.

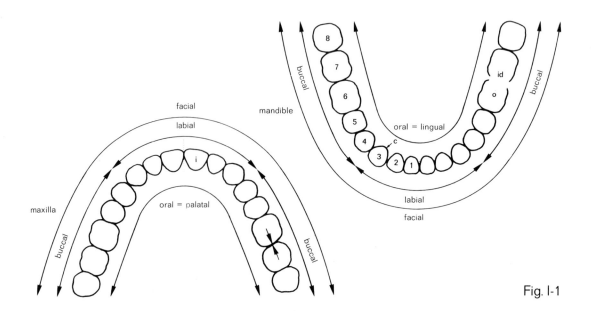

Fig. I-1

Distal = away from the midline

Mesial = towards the midline

Facial = That aspect of a tooth which faces, or is in contact with, the cheek or lip mucosa. This is a general term; more specificity may be achieved by using the terms "buccal," meaning toward the cheek, and "labial," meaning toward the lip.

Oral   = that aspect of a tooth which faces, or is in contact with, the tongue or palate. More specifically, "lingual" means toward the tongue and "palatal" signifies toward the palate, though "lingual" (but not "palatal") is a term often used synonomously with "oral."

id   = interdental (between the teeth)

i   = incisal, biting edge

o   = occlusal, chewing surface

c   = cervical (at the neck of the tooth)

The surfaces of two adjacent teeth which touch each other are referred to as "proximal" surfaces (→←).

40

Positioning the Patient in the Treatment Chair

1. Seated patient (conventional position)

Adjust the back of the chair and the headrest for comfortable, relaxed sitting. Vary chair height for examination and treatment in the maxilla (Max) and mandible (Mand), oral or facial aspects.

The position of the patient should be adjusted to conform to the body position of the dentist - and not vice versa. Correct standing posture = upright position. Do not maintain a forced position for extended periods of time; avoid acrobatic contortions.

For examination with **direct** lighting, the following sitting position of the patient has proven useful for the beginner:

Max: Relatively high chair position with a slightly backward tilting of the chair. Patient's head and operator's eyes should be at about the same height.

Mand: Lower chair position. The operator's chin should be at the same height as the top of the patient's head. With a seated patient, the occlusal plane to be examined should be horizontal.

Planes of orientation in the cranial region (see Fig. I-2).

Camper plane:

This is an imaginary line connecting subnasion and the center of the external auditory meatus.

Frankfurt horizontal:

Line connecting the superior margin of the external auditory meatus (tragion) to the most caudal point of the orbital margin (orbitale).

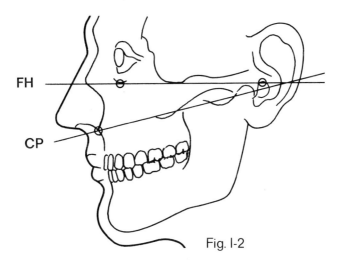

Fig. I-2

2. Reclining patient

Learning *sit-down* dentistry represents one facet of what is called "ergonomic centistry."[1] In recent years, treatment performed with the patient in a reclining position has become commonplace in the dental office. The literature in the field of ergonomics (= conservation of energy) is enormous.

A Central Institute for Dental Ergonomics is located in Coblenz, West Germany.

In the reclining position, the patient's legs are positioned quite high. It is a relaxed position. The dentist sits upright; work is performed with a chairside dental assistant ("four-handed dentistry"); a high speed evacuator is used; direct vision is possible in both maxilla and mandible; treatment time can be lengthened.

Irony and Ergonomics (I):

My two legs are no longer weary!
My varicose veins are gone, nearly!
But filled is the plexus
Right near the sexus
And of that my patients are leery!

Irony and Ergonomics (II).

My two legs no longer have pain!
Gone is my varicose vein!
But, you see, its no riddle
Where blood pools near my middle.
From sitting I'll have to refrain!

[1] Good introduction in "Die Quintessenz," special edition "Ergonomie," vol. 17, October, 1966. The latest publications may be found (primarily in the German literature) under the names F. Schön and K. H. Kimmel.
In addition:
Weinert, A. M.: An evaluation of the modern dental lounge chair. Dent. Clinics N. A. 15, 129 – 155; 1971.
Recent publication: Kimmel, K., Walker, R. O.: Practising Dentistry, Ergonomic Guidelines for the Future. Verlag "Die Quintessenz" Publishers, Berlin and Chicago, 1972.

Lighting

Lux = the unit of measurement for light intensity = light current density = number of lumens per surface area. The illumination of the oral cavity attained with various operatinglight sources (e. g., Luminaire, Two-Field lighting, Miralux, halogen lamp, fiber optics) may be quite different.
Room lighting should be 600 lux; the immediate vicinity of the operating chair, 600 to 1,000 lux; the patient's head, 1,000 lux; the mouth, 8,000 to 13,000 lux[3]; a fiber optic tip, 24,000 lux.
Direct lighting without a mirror is called "direct vision."
Indirect lighting with a mirror = "indirect vision." Some disadvantages of this method include clouding of the mirror by the spray and by drill dust, and fogging of the mirror by the patient's exhalations.

Transillumination

Transillumination involves use of a fiberoptic apparatus to look "through" oral structures. It is a procedure best performed in a darkened room. Alterations in enamel and dentin often appear then as opaque, dark areas. The apical region can also be checked by this means. It may be possible to detect pulpal necrosis as well.

The fiberoptic light source[1,2]

Light is transmitted by bundles of glass fibers, which provide total reflection at the glass surface. Because of the rate of loss of light intensity with distance, a strong light source such as a cooled halogen lamp is required.

Use of the fiberoptic apparatus

There are many potential uses for the fiberoptic apparatus in the dental treatment area. Some of these include:
1. transillumination of all parts of the mouth for identification of abnormalities, e. g., dental caries
2. obtaining good illumination for treatment in distal areas of the mouth, or where access is limited
3. searching for root canals
4. as an aid in location and removal of broken root canal instruments
5. during surgical operations.

In the future, a fiberoptic apparatus will no doubt be routinely built into dental units.

[1] Friedmann, J., Marcus, M. I.: Transillumination of the oral cavity with use of fiber optics. J.A.D.A. 80, 801; 1970.
[2] Büchs, H.: Der flexible Lichtleiter. Dtsch. Zahnärztebl. 24, 18; 1970.
[3] DIN 67505: Beleuchtung zahnärztlicher Arbeitsstätten. Benth-Vertrieb GmbH, Berlin W15, 1962.
[4] Riedel, H.: Der Arbeitsplatz. Praxis der Zahnheilkunde. Volume I A–Z. Urban & Schwarzenberg, Munich, 1969.

The Clinical Treatment Area

Subject: _____

Examiner: _____

Date: _____

1. Identify the various handles and buttons for adjustment of treatment chair height, seat back position and head rest.   Completion   ☐

2. With the patient seated comfortably, adjust the headrest for examination in the maxilla.   Completion   ☐

3. Do the same for examination in the mandible.   Completion   ☐

4. Position the head of a comfortably seated patient so that the following landmarks are horizontal:

   a) Camper plane   Completion   ☐

   b) Frankfurt horizontal   Completion   ☐

5. What is the position of the maxillary occlusal plane relative to the true horizontal when:

   a) the patient's head is positioned as in 4a (above)   cranial   post. _____ ant.

   b) the patient's head is positioned as in 4b (above)   post. _____ ant.   caudal

(In the space below, draw in the position of the occlusal plane with the approximate angle. Use your protractor.)

6. Transilluminate the upper anterior teeth, first with direct
   light and then using fiberoptics.   Completion   ☐

7. Position the patient for examination:

   by a standing dentist

   a) with direct vision of the lingual surface of tooth 42   Completion   ☐

   b) with indirect vision of the lingual surface of 42   Completion   ☐

   by a seated dentist

   c) with direct vision of the palatal surface of tooth 16   Completion   ☐

   d) with indirect vision of the lingual surface of 46   Completion   ☐

Instructor's signature: _____

Operatory Hygiene

Instruction Sheets

II-1: Hygiene at the treatment chair
II-2: Demonstration of bacteria

Exercise and Data Sheet

II-2: Demonstration of bacteria

Material

Student: clinic kit

Instructor: items for bacteriological exercises; media, filters etc.

Program

1. General introduction
2. Introduction to today's topic
3. Demonstration of bacteria

Demonstrations

1. Air investigations
    a) investigation of room air by exposure of medium in petri dishes
    b) slit sampler

2. Water investigation with membrane filter method
    a) tap water
    b) demineralized water
    c) water from air turbine handpiece reservoir

3. Reduction of bacterial count by hand washing and hand disinfection

4. Microbiological samples taken from bracket table, instruments, handles and beard

5. Analysis of the sterility of the clinic kit

Hygiene at the Treatment Chair

In addition to the need to maintain the best possible personal hygiene, we must also sustain a high level of hygiene around the treatment chair and in the operatory at large, in order to prevent disease transmission from one patient to another. Furthermore, correct hygiene provides both dentist and operatory personnel with the optimum level of protection against infection.

Contamination may occur in a dental practice in the following ways (among others):

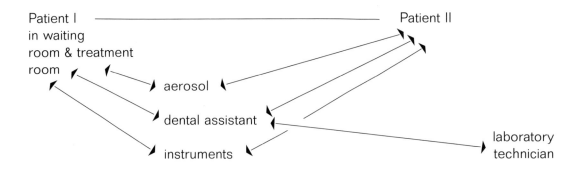

Patients, dentist, dental assistant and the laboratory technician may contaminate each other with bacteria. They may do this through actual personal contact or by way of instruments. Indirectly, airborne contamination within the treatment room or, more rarely, within the waiting room, is also possible. Pathogenic microorganisms may remain on impressions, on partially completed prosthetic appliances or trays, and even on the impression trays. In all such instances they present a danger of infection to the dental technician. Conversely, microorganisms from the technician may infect the patient.

The possibilities of contamination through direct contact are readily imagined (person, instruments, table top, air syringe, water spray tip). Most *contact infection* can be avoided if one autoclaves all sterilizable instruments, and carefully disinfects non-sterilizable materials, such as the various impression materials.

Careful *hand washing* is the first step in reducing the number of microorganisms. However, washing alone does not free the hands completely of microorganisms. The reusable cloth towel has to be considered a "bacterial playground." Use absorbant disposable towels! Or cotton toweling on a roll! Again, after you shake hands with a patient, wash your hands!

Impression materials can be disinfected with UV light (UV box).

Use of the high speed handpiece with water spray creates several possibilities for the dissemination of bacteria, e. g.:

a) Spraying out bacteria which are present in the coolant water
At least two types of organisms have been isolated from air turbine water (Ps. aerogenes and Alcaligenes faecalis). The number of microorganisms, that is, the extent of the contamination, will be determined by the bacteriological situation in the water softening apparatus and in the air turbine itself, as well as by the length of time the water has remained in the reservoir and in the lines.[1] Regular disinfection of water lines, and the use of sterilized, distilled water are absolutely essential. Water from a softening apparatus must be checked for bacterial content on a regular basis.

b) Dissemination of bacteria and viruses from the patient's mouth
Tiny contaminated water particles, because of their light weight, remain suspended in the air as an aerosol for a long time. When they finally settle upon equipment and/or instruments, contamination results.

Intraoral use of the water spray immediately produces such an aerosol, which exposes both the dentist and the chairside assistant to infection by the patient's microorganisms. In addition, when this aerosol finally settles upon equipment or instruments, another form of potential contamination results.

Although most dentists are aware of the danger of patient-to-patient bacterial contamination due to inadequate disinfection of the handpiece, they are inclined to take the danger of aerosol transmission of microorganisms far too lightly.

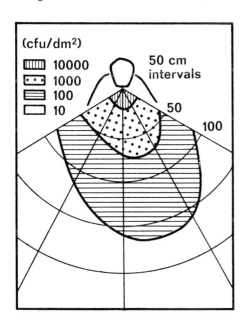

In Figure II-1, the dissemination of microorganisms after a 30-second use of the water-cooled air turbine handpiece is depicted as "colony forming units" (cfu) per dm². One sees that even 1.50 meters from the oral cavity, there is still contamination at the level of 100 cfu.

See R. L. Miller[2] for details about "dental aerobiology."

In the future, the treatment room will be equipped with special air conditioning for removal of aerosols (principle of vertical laminar air streaming).

Fig. II-1

[1] Translator's note: Most high speed handpieces in the United States are cooled by water taken directly from the community water supply line. This water is assumed to be reasonably safe for intraoral use.
[2] Miller, R. L. et al.: J. dent. Res. 48, 49 1969. – J. dent. Res. 50, 621; 1971. – J. dent. Res. 50, 626; 1971.

The dentist cannot avoid aerosols, yet his risk of infection is reduced if he wears a mask and protective glasses. The danger of infection for the patient can be reduced by the dentist's frequent changing of his outer garments (clinic gown or jacket) and through the regular disinfection of all surfaces where instruments or materials may be placed.

Prevention

The concentration of viable bacteria in the aerosol can be reduced by 90% if, before the intraoral procedure is begun, the patient rinses 3 times for 10 seconds with 20 ml of an antiseptic mouthwash (chlorhexidine, 0.2 %[1,2]), or when the teeth are brushed with a chlorhexidine-containing gel! Don't forget it!

Bearded students will be interested in the extent to which microorganisms caught within the aerosol are trapped by beard hair, posing the danger of transmission to other patients and personnel. If you wear a beard, do not let your patients read the article by *Pollock*[3]... !

The Bearded Dentist:

> There once was a dentist from Biel,
> Who washed himself often with zeal.
> But though properly reared,
> Because of his beard
> He was never completely sterile . . .

Literature

Grün, L. und Crott, K.: Ueber den Keimgehalt des Turbinensprays. I. Fahrbare Turbinen. DZZ 24, 189; 1969.

Grün, L. und Crott, K.: Ueber den Keimgehalt des Turbinensprays. II. Eingebaute Turbinen. DZZ 24, 870; 1969.

Editorial. Cross Infection in General Dental Practice. Int. Dent. J. 15, 393; 1965.

Grün, L.: Probleme der Desinfektion in zahnärztlichem Bereich. DZZ 22, 1169–1175; 1967.

Engelhardt, J. P.: Experimentelle Untersuchungen über die Desinfektion. DZZ 22, 1175–1183; 1967.

Bauer, E., Langer, H., Portelle, K.: Turbine und Keimstreuung. DZZ, 1183–1196; 1967.

Fuhr, K.: Klinische und experimentelle Untersuchungen zur Desinfektion und Sterilisation. DZZ 22, 1196–1205; 1967.

Pollock, N. L., Shay, D. E., Williams, G. H.: Evaluation of airborne contamination in a dental school clinic. J. Baltimore Coll. Dent. Surg. 27, 1; 1973.

Miller, R. L., Micik, R. E., Abel, D., Ryge, G.: Studies on dental aerobiology: II. Microbial splatter discharged from the oral cavity of dental patients. J. Dent. Res. 50, 621; 1971.

[1] Translator's note: While chlorhexidine is employed routinely in continental Europe and in Scandinavia, Federal regulations still prohibit its use in the United States.

[2] Wyler, D., Miller, R. L., Micik, R. E.: Efficiency of self-administered preoperative oral hygiene procedures in reducing the concentration of bacteria in aerosols generated during dental procedures. J. dent. Res. 50, 509; 1971.

[3] Pollock, N. L. et al.: Airborne contamination of beards by dental aerosols. 48th General Meeting I.A.D.R., New York, 1970, and J. Baltimore College Dental Surgery, 1971.

Demonstration of Bacteria

1. Airborne bacteria

Simple plate exposure

We know that germs in the air sink in response to gravity. Culture medium in a petri dish is exposed to the air for 15 to 60 minutes. Bacteria which fall onto the medium will become visible after incubation as colonies, which can be counted.

This method gives only a rough estimate of the degree of air contamination by bacteria. Air currents, of course, affect the results.

Greenburg-Smith Impinger

The air to be examined is pulled through a liquid with the help of a pump (impingement). This is a good procedure if one does not know what contaminants to expect, because various substrates can be employed. The impingers are first sterilized with 150 ml of phosphate buffer solution (pH 7.0). In order to insure that the bacteria are actually taken up, two impingers are placed one after the other. To prevent bacterial overgrowth during the experiment, impingers are cooled to 3-4° C. Air is pulled through at the rate of 25 liters per minute. Aliquots are subjected to the usual microbiologic procedures. The bacterial counts obtained are then expressed as the number of bacteria per cubic meter of air. Membrane filter methods may also be considered (see Section 2., Waterborne bacteria).

Impaction sampler

This is a "collision" procedure for the sampling of air. The air to be examined is pulled through a narrow orifice, causing acceleration of the various bacterial carriers in the air (dust, pollen, water vapor). These collide with a culture medium surface and remain. The Andersen Sampler permits additional separation according to the size of the bacterial carrier. With the slit sampler, 29 liters of air per minute are pulled through a 0.3 mm wide, 28 mm long slit. This air is blown directly onto a 90 mm diameter culture plate, the surface of which is 2 mm beneath the slit. The culture plate is rotated continuously during the time that the air sample is being collected; the speed of rotation can be varied. It is possible to make statements concerning changes in germ concentration during the course of the sample collection. Furthermore, total germ counts may be determined, in cubic meter units.

The bacterial counts per m^3 of air vary approximately as follows:

Outside air	100 – 50,000
Air within te Federal Institute of Technology	9,810
Air within a dental office	1,000 – 100,000

Air within a dental school demonstration room during a treatment procedure   88,375
Air within other office areas   100 – 15,000

2. Waterborne bacteria

Quantitative analysis

One milliliter of H_2O is serially diluted by a factor of ten. One milliliter of an indicated dilution is pipetted into a sterile petri dish, covered with melted agar (50° C) and mixed well. After incubation, the colonies are counted.

Membrane filter method

500 ml of H_2O are pulled through a membrane filter with a pore size of 0.45 μm. The membrane filter is then transferred by means of sterile forceps to an appropriate culture medium, and incubated. During the incubation, the trapped bacteria grow into countable colonies, because the nutrients from the culture plate surface diffuse through the pores.

Note:

The choice of culture medium is an important determinant for test results. The medium is selected according to the type of contamination suspected. Endoagar will be used, for example, in the case of enterobacteria. For our demonstration in the operatory, only sheep blood plates will be employed, because we are primarily interested in oral microorganisms.

The germ counts per milliliter of water vary approximately as follows:

Well water (from the Sihl-Lorze region of Switzerland)	0 – 100
Lake water	40 – 15,000
Limmat River, Zurich	4,000 – 90,000
Filtered lake water	3 – 38
Water demineralized with resin	$100 - 10^6$
x̄ from 27 dental offices	87,000*

Drinking water which has met the latest Swiss governmental
standards   200 coliform organisms

---

* Studies on dental aerobiology: IV Bacterial contamination of water delivered by dental units, J. Dent. Res., 50, 1567–1574; 1971.

Odiferous drills:

An air turbine drill truly stank.
Bacteria swam in the tank.
Rid water and lines
Of germs and of slimes!
Your patients will surely say "Thanks"!

Demonstration of Bacteria*

1. Determine the number of colonies after simple culture medium exposure within the clinic

Plate No.	Location	Exposure time (min)	Number of colonies
Plate 1			
Plate 2			
Plate 3			

2. Slit sampler

On the basis of the number of visible colonies, calculate the bacterial counts per m³ of air in the laboratory. Time = 5 min. Pump setting = 28 L. of air per minute.

3. Water investigation using membrane filter method

Estimate the germ counts per liter

– in tap water _____

– in distilled water _____

– in water from the air turbine tank _____

4. According to the results of our investigations, which method of drying the hands should be recommended?

5. Observe the work of the dental assistant in the clinic, keeping in mind the results of plate streakings from various surfaces.

6. Was your personal clinic kit shown to be sterile?

* This demonstration should be performed by the instructor.

Orofacial Examination

Instruction Sheet

III-1: Oral Examination

Exercise and Data Sheets

III-1 Extraoral Examination

III-2: Mandibular movements

Results Sheet

III-1: Mandibular movements

Material

Student: clinic kit, colored pencils, grease pencil, compass

Instructor: stethoscope, millimeter measuring strips, gauze squares

Program

1. Demonstration of the microbiological results from Exercise II

2. Discussion of today's topic

3. Exercises in groups of 2 to 3 students

   a) Performance of "extraoral examination" and completing data sheets

   b) Measuring mandibular movements; auscultation of the temporomandibular joint

The experienced clinician will begin to evaluate the general physical condition of the patient as soon as he enters the operatory. With experience, a patient can usually be categorized at first glance as "completely healthy," "perhaps healthy," "probably sick" or "sick." In a beginning course, however, this type of medical insight cannot be expected.

Extraoral Examination

In any type of examination, a step-by-step procedure must be followed. Not to do so invites consequences which can be both embarrassing for the dentist and dangerous for the patient, if early symptoms of serious disease go undected.

During the physical examination, the practitioner uses his various *senses* to check the patient.

Vision

The eye inspects. Visual inspection includes a search for changes in the *color* and *shape* of tissues, as well as an observation of patient *movements*. In this connection, left-right symmetry is especially important.

Examples

1. Slight swelling in the right submandibular region. Is this due to lymph node enlargement, to salivary gland swelling, or to something else?

2. A scarcely visible reddening of the left cheek. Does this indicate a skin disorder or a pathological condition in the subjacent bone?

3. An asymmetric opening movement of the lower jaw, with deviation to the left. Is some disorder of the temporomandibular joint causing this functional manifestation?

Touch

The sense of touch is employed to detect alterations in the consistency and mobility of tissues. For example, there is normally a degree of mobility between the skin and its underlying (muscular and osseous) structures. The sense of touch should be used to detect any increase or decrease in this degree of mobility, wherever possible. More specifically, the cheeks and the floor of the mouth should be palpated bidigitally (= with two fingers), with one finger outside the mouth and the other inside the oral cavity.

Palpation is especially important in areas where abnormalities of color and shape have been noticed.

Remember that the skin on the back of your hand is very sensitive, a fact which can be of use in detection of temperature abnormalities.

In many cases, your palpation will cause the patient some discomfort. You should note carefully the patient's reaction to pressure applied upon and around swollen, reddened or other abnormal areas.

Examples:

1. A firm nodule beneath the skin yet adherent to it, in the submandibular region.

2. No alterations in skin consistency, but sensitivity to pressure applied in the area overlying the infraorbital foramen, where the second division of the trigeminal nerve exits the cranium.

3. A stone-hard growth detected during bidigital palpation of the floor of the mouth.

4. Reduced air flow from the left nostril, detected by relative amounts of fogging of a cold mirror held next to the separate nostrils (The difference in temperature between warm air and the cold mirror surface make this possible).

Hearing

Through the trained sense of hearing, we can detect sounds which occur during palpation, percussion and during movements of body parts.

Examples:

1. Crepitus of a swelling at the right mandibular angle subsequent to extraction of the third molar tooth. Air emphysema?

2. A dull sound evident upon percussion of a tooth (compare left and right sides!). Could this be due to periodontitis, or to a non-vital tooth?

3. A "popping" of the right temporomandibular joint during opening, with simultaneous deviation to the left.

Olfaction

The sense of smell enables one to detect the odor of the patient's breath as well as body odor. One must determine if the odor is systemic in origin, for example the fruity smell of diabetes mellitus, or something localized to a source in the mouth or the nose (e. g., tonsillitis, periodontal pockets, sinusitis).

We're resigned to *not* using our sense of *taste* . . .!

In order not to forget anything while we are performing an extraoral examination of the head region, it is important after initial inspection and palpation to check the functions of the most important cranial nerves. Things to be reviewed include:

a. Symmetry or asymmetry of the pupils
b. Pupil reaction to light
c. Symmetrical or asymmetrical movements of the muscles of facial expression:
    wrinkling the forehead
    opening the eyes
    whistling
    laughing

d. Normal sensitivity of facial skin. Hypo- and paraesthesia
e. Pain upon palpation of infraorbital foramen
f. Pain upon palpation of the temporomandibular joint.

Eye symmetry:

> A girl observed sensitively
> Her lack of true eye symmetry.
> But she'd plenty of bread
> And wore contacts instead
> Of horn-rimmed optometry!

Intraoral Examination

The practitioner must lay down for himself an absolute rule: Before examining the dentition, always inspect the entire oral cavity and the throat region in a good light, and palpate wherever possible. Nobody dies from a toothache, but early malignancies are all too often overlooked in the oral cavity. Examine your patient in the same way you yourself would want to be examined!

Always follow the same pattern, combining inspection with palpation, and comparing the left side to the right side.

1. Pharynx-palate

Have the patient say "aaaah." What about the color, shape and symmetry of the isthmus of fauces? How large are the tonsils? Are the tonsillar surfaces normal?

2. Tongue and floor of the mouth

a) Palpate the floor of the mouth with both hands, one finger inside the mouth and the other hand outside and supporting the mandible.
b) Have the patient lick both right and left corners of the mouth. Is the tongue clean, or coated? Check size, positon, color and moblity of the tongue. Is the tongue symmetrical when it is protruded?

3. Cheek mucosa

Are Fordyce's granules present? Are there other mucosal alterations? Can you see any pigmentation of the mucosa? It is imperative to palpate the oral vestibulum; have the patient close slightly for palpation of the maxillary vestibule's canine fossae and tuberosity regions. Also, palpate the retromolar areas in both maxilla and mandible.

4. Salivary gland function

a) Review this by "milking" the parotid gland while observing the dried intraoral ductal opening, and then by
b) extraoral palpation of the submandibular gland with simultaneous observation of the ductal openings along the floor of the mouth.

5. Taste disturbances.

Does the patient report a metallic taste? Is there evidence of hypo- or paraesthesia of the tongue?

6. Saliva

We will discuss saliva in a subsequent exercise.

Literature

Brachmann, F.: Die Zahnärztliche Untersuchung. Praxis der Zahnheilkunde, Vol. I., Urban and Schwarzenberg, Munich, 1970.

Extraoral Examination

Subject: _____

Examiner: _____

Date: _____

Answer the following questions by checking the proper box.

		Yes	No
1. Are eye pupils symmetrical?		☐	☐
2. Is there obvious pupillary contraction when exposed to light?	left right	☐ ☐	☐ ☐
3. Is eyelid opening symmetrical?		☐	☐
4. Symmetrical forehead wrinkling?		☐	☐
5. Is the mouth symmetrical during whistling?		☐	☐
6. Is the mouth symmetrical during laughing?		☐	☐
7. Is skin sensitivity similar on left and right sides of forehead? cheek? submental triangle?		☐ ☐ ☐	☐ ☐ ☐
8. Is nasal breathing normal?	left right	☐ ☐	☐ ☐
9. Are there palpable submandibular lymph nodes?	left right	☐ ☐	☐ ☐
10. Sensitivity of Valleix pressure points I, II, III?	left right	☐ ☐	☐ ☐

Instructor's signature: _____

Mandibular Movements

Make the following measurements using your compass* and enter all data on Data Sheet III-2. While making these measurements, always palpate the head of the mandibular condyle simultaneously.

1. Measure in millimeters the maximum mandibular opening.

Procedure:

This distance is the sum of

a) interincisal distance (i) and
b) amount of overbite (o) (this measurement may be a negative figure in cases of open bite)

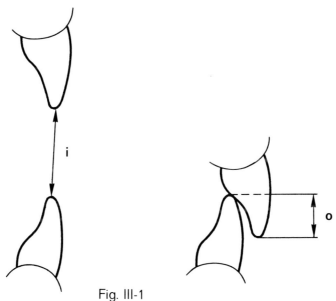

Fig. III-1

2. Measure in millimeters the maximum lateral mandibular excursion during occlusal contact.

Procedure:

Mark with a grease pencil on the labial surface of the maxillary anterior teeth the position of the interdental space between 31 and 41 (m)

---

* Translator's note: To use the compass, for example to measure distance "i" in the Figure above, place the tip of one compass arm at the incisal edge of the upper incisor, and the other tip at incisal edge of the mandibular tooth. Then measure the distance between the compass arm tips with a millimeter rule.

a) in habitual occlusion (maximum interdigitation)

Fig. III-2
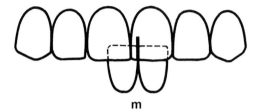

m

b) in the maximum lateral excursion to the left (ml) and then right (mr)

Fig. III-3
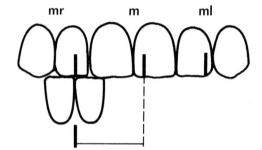

mr   m   ml

maximum excursion to right

3. Auscultate with the stethoscope both temporomandibular joints during the three phases of the mandibular opening movement. Are any unusual sounds detectable? Enter what you hear and when you hear any sound such as popping (P), friction (F), or other noises (N).

4. Observe the mandibular midline during opening. Is there lateral deviation? Make a sketch of what you see.

Mandibular Movements

Subject: _____

Examiner: _____

Date: _____

1. Measurement of maximum mandibular opening

    Inter-incisal distance (i)   _____ mm
    Overbite   (o)   _____ mm
    Total opening   (i + o)   _____ mm

2. Measurement of maximum mandibular lateral excursion

    to the left   _____ mm
    to the right   _____ mm

3. Auscultation of the TMJ during opening. Insert P, F, or N, as appropriate. Put a line through the space if no sounds are heard.

left   right

		left	right
"Popping",	initial phase of opening		
Friction	intermediate phase		
other noises	terminal phase		
	continuous		

4. Draw a line to show movement of the mandible in the frontal plane during opening

beginning movement

maximal opening
(the line shown here is an
example of opening *without*
deviation)

5. Hand in the signed result sheet.

Instructor's signature: _____

Mandibular Movements

1. The following measurements were made on 28 subjects in a previous exercise. Data are given in millimeters:

	average	range
Maximum interincisal distance	52.7 ± 8.4	39 – 69 mm
Overbite	4.3 ± 2.0	1 – 8
Maximum mandibular opening	57.0 ± 8.4	43 – 73

Open and eat:

> Said the Professor: "To me its no riddle
> How students eat lots, not a little.
> The reason, no doubt,
> Is the great open mouth
> Which is ever so wide in the middle"!

A Japanese study[1] reported maximum mandibular opening to be 43.4 mm. Lateral excursive movement to the left was 14.2 mm; to the right, 12.3 mm.

2. In the same 28 subjects, the maximum lateral movement of the mandible was:

	average	range
a) to the left	11.8 ± 5.2	6 – 32 mm
b) to the right	11.7 ± 5.1	5 – 30

The range of lateral excursion is an important thing to note. In extreme cases it may be no greater than 5 or 6 mm. Is this because of a functional disturbance (spasticity) of the masticatory musculature or is it caused by an anatomical hindrance? Check for symmetry!

3. In 56 temporomandibular joints of 28 subjects, abnormal noises were detected with the following frequency:

initial phase of opening	7 times
intermediate phase	10 times
terminal phase	4 times

[1] Bull. Tokyo Med. Dent. Univ. 16, 123; 1969.

Radiology

Instruction Sheets

IV-1: Radiographic technique
IV-2: Radiographic caries diagnosis

Exercise and Data Sheets

IV-1: Radiographic technique
IV-2: Radiographic caries diagnosis

Material

Student: clinic set, impression tray. Personal radiographic survey. Red pencil.

Instructor: x-ray viewboxes, dental radiographs, bite-wing films for caries diagnosis.
           Impression materials.

Program

1. Discussion of the results from Exercise III (Result Sheet III-1)

2. Introduction to radiographic caries diagnosis

3. Demonstration of radiographic technique

4. Exercises in caries diagnosis

5. Impression-taking by students of each other

Division of the entire class into 4 groups for demonstrations and exercises. These groups rotate every 25 minutes.

Radiographic Technique

X-ray machine

The most important elements of an x-ray machine are: cathode, anode, filter, shutter. The path taken by the central ray, as well as dispersion and extraneous rays must also be considered.

X-ray film

X-ray film consists of: paper covering, protective layer, 2 films (coated on both sides), lead foil.

Radiographic theory

X-rays are absorbed to varying degrees by different tissues. The photosensitive layer on the film is altered to greater or lesser extent, depending upon the quantity of x-rays which penetrate the tissue. We may differentiate between "hard" (short wave length) and "soft" (long wave length) x-rays. Voltage (kV), current (mA) and exposure time are critical factors when taking radiographs.

The bisecting-angle technique

Because of anatomical restrictions, the intraoral film (30 x 40 mm) is not placed parallel to the object (tooth long axis). The central ray is directed along a line which bisects the planes of the film and the long axis of the tooth. With the film in this position, minimal distortion of the object results. Indications for the bisecting angle technique include endodontics and radiography of edentulous spaces. Sharpness of the picture can be improved by increasing the distance between x-ray source and object (long-cone technique).

Parallel technique

In this technique the intraoral film (30 x 40 mm) is placed parallel to the object (tooth long axis) using a special film-holding apparatus. The central ray is directed perpendicularly to both film and object. If the long-cone technique is employed, almost perfect image size and shape may be obtained. Film holders may also be useful for exact duplication of a radiograph (standardized radiographic technique for reproducible films). Indication for the parallel technique: periodontology. Cotton rolls may be used in the absence of a film-holding apparatus to achieve pretty good parallel results.

Bitewing technique

The somewhat longer (e. g., 27 x 54 mm) bitewing film is held in place by having the patient bite together onto the film tab. Both maxillary and mandibular bicuspid and molar tooth crowns are radiographed simultaneously. To reduce overlapping in the inter-dental areas, the long-cone technique is employed. Indications for bitewing technique: diagnosis of carious lesions in young people; to check margins of crowns and fillings; depiction of proximal dental calculus (or even heavy labial or lingual calculus).

Recommended literature:

Mourshed, F., McKinney, A. L.: A comparison of paralleling and bisecting radiographic techniques as experienced by dental students. Oral Surg. 33, 284; 1972.

Stafne, E. C.: Röntgendiagnostik des Mundes und der Zähne mit einem Anhang über Röntgen-technik. Media-Verlag, Stuttgart, 3. Auflage, 1971.

Radiographic Technique

Subject: _____

Examiner: _____

Date: _____

Answer the following questions by checking the appropriate spaces:

	True	False
1. The central ray courses from cathode to anode.	_____	_____
2. The light areas on the radiograph (negative) are radiolucent.	_____	_____
3. In the bisecting angle technique, the central ray is directed perpendicular to a line which bisects the angle between facial skin and tooth long axis.	_____	_____
4. The bitewing radiograph is most useful for depiction of proximal carious lesions in the anterior teeth.	_____	_____
5. Enamel is more radiopaque than dentin.	_____	_____
6. Short wave rays reduce the radiopacity.	_____	_____
7. In Grade 1 radiographic proximal caries, the radiolucency extends only to the dentoenamel junction.	_____	_____
8. Chalky spots on facial tooth surfaces are not visible on the bitewing radiograph.	_____	_____
9. Wedge-shaped cervical defects are always visible on the radiograph.	_____	_____
10. Careful examination of proximal carious lesions with mirror, explorer and good lighting is not better than radiographic examination.	_____	_____

Instructor's signature: _____

Radiographic Caries Diagnosis

1. Material

Bitewing radiographs for simultaneous depiction of posterior tooth crowns in maxilla and mandible.
Periapical radiographs: large for posterior teeth, small for anterior teeth.

2. Terminology

The radiograph is a two-dimensional light-dark picture. It is always the negative which is observed and evaluated.

Radiopaque = structures which do not permit the passage of x-rays; the film is therefore exposed incompletely (if at all). Transparent, light areas on the radiographic negative are caused by radiopaque structures.

Radiolucent = structures which permit the passage of x-rays, yet offer some resistance; the film is therefore heavily exposed. Dark, or even black, areas on the radiographic negative are caused by radiolucent structures.

3. Differentiation among radiopacities

Complete opacity is caused by metals, e. g., silver amalgam or gold fillings.

Strong opacity is caused by enamel, due to its dense structure and high mineral content (98%).

Medium opacity is caused by less dense structures such as dentin and dental calculus. Mineral content of dentin is 75%, of calculus 50 – 75%, depending on its age.
The opacity caused by osseous tissue (mineral content 65%) depends essentially upon bony structure. A strong opacity is occasioned by the thick cortical bone and a weaker one by areas of cancellous bone. For example, the cortical bone inside the dental alveolus is a clearly visible radiopaque structure, called the *lamina dura*.

Weak opacity is caused by the dental pulp, the periodontal ligament and by bone marrow.

4. Caries diagnosis

Because of demineralization, radiolucencies become apparent in the normally radiopaque enamel and dentin.

Radiographic classification of proximal lesions:

Grade 1 Wedge-shaped radiolucency in the outermost enamel layer (chalky spot)

Grade 2 Radiolucency also extends into the inner enamel layer (chalky spot or initial defect)

Grade 3 Earliest evidence of cone-shaped radiolucency in the dentin beneath the enamel (This represents a certain defect)

Grade 4 Radiolucency extends into deeper dentin layers (carious defect, carious cavity)

Occlusal and smooth surface carious lesions are visible on the radiography only when they are very deep.

Root caries may be observed below the radiographically evident proximal cemento-enamel junction. These lesions are usually wide, not generally very deep, and can only be seen on the radiograph when located proximally. It is easy to mistake them for artefacts.

Differential diagnosis of carious lesions:

Enamel opacities, enamel fluorosis: not visible radiographically.

Enamel hypoplasia: only visible if very large; light area.

Enamel erosion: seldom detectable on the radiograph.

Wedge-shaped cervical defects (e. g., toothbrush abrasion): if severe, seen as a radio-lucency.

With bitewing radiographs, 20–100% more carious lesions of proximal surfaces of posterior teeth can be detected than with the use of mirror and explorer alone. But the x-ray doesn't see *everything* either! 70% of initial carious lesions cannot be detected on the bitewing radiograph, even though clinically (on the extracted tooth) a chalky spot or even a microdefect is already present. The radiographic picture lags behind the actual microscopic situation. The radiographic latent period for lytic alterations (resorption) of bone is about 3 weeks; for demineralization of enamel (chalky spot formation), it averages about 6 months.

Dangerous rays:

"This machine," the technician says,
"Produces mysterious rays,
    Which permit detection
    But wear your protection
Or you'll go eaten up to your grave."

Radiographic Caries Diagnosis

Subject: _____

Bitewing film No. _____

Date: _____

Material

Two bitewing radiographs, left and right, will be provided. Each student should bring his own personal radiographic survey. An x-ray viewbox is also required.

Bitewing films

1. Circle permanent teeth which are unerupted.

18 17 16 15 14 13 12 11	21 22 23 24 25 26 27 28
48 47 46 45 44 43 42 41	31 32 33 34 35 36 37 38

2. Cross out permanent teeth which cannot be evaluated.

18 17 16 15 14 13 12 11	21 22 23 24 25 26 27 28
48 47 46 45 44 43 42 41	31 32 33 34 35 36 37 38

3. At the bottom of page 72, sketch what you observed on the right bitewing radiograph. Include enamel, dentin, carious radiolucencies, radiopaque fillings, etc. Score the proximal surfaces which have caries with Grades 1, 2, 3 or 4.

Personal radiographic survey

1. Circle all teeth which have been extracted (6)* or which are unerupted (7)*.
How many teeth are erupted? ☐

18 17 16 15 14 13 12 11	21 22 23 24 25 26 27 28
48 47 46 45 44 43 42 41	31 32 33 34 35 36 37 38

2. Circle all teeth which have metal fillings.
How many have none? ☐

18 17 16 15 14 13 12 11	21 22 23 24 25 26 27 28
48 47 46 45 44 43 42 41	31 32 33 34 35 36 37 38

* Mark with a 6 (6 = extracted) or a 7 (7 = remaining).

3. Circle teeth which have
non-metallic fillings.
How many have none? ☐

18 17 16 15 14 13 12 11	21 22 23 24 25 26 27 28
48 47 46 45 44 43 42 41	31 32 33 34 35 36 37 38

4. Circle teeth which are
probably nonvital.
How many
are probably vital? ☐

18 17 16 15 14 13 12 11	21 22 23 24 25 26 27 28
48 47 46 45 44 43 42 41	31 32 33 34 35 36 37 38

5. Circle all proximal surfaces
which have untreated carious
enamel lesions of Grades 1
and 2.

18 17 16 15 14 13 12 11	21 22 23 24 25 26 27 28
48 47 46 45 44 43 42 41	31 32 33 34 35 36 37 38

6. Circle teeth which have
untreated carious dentin lesions
of Grades 3 and 4.

18 17 16 15 14 13 12 11	21 22 23 24 25 26 27 28
48 47 46 45 44 43 42 41	31 32 33 34 35 36 37 38

7. Circle teeth which have
carious secondary lesions.

18 17 16 15 14 13 12 11	21 22 23 24 25 26 27 28
48 47 46 45 44 43 42 41	31 32 33 34 35 36 37 38

8. Circle teeth which have
detectable calculus.

18 17 16 15 14 13 12 11	21 22 23 24 25 26 27 28
48 47 46 45 44 43 42 41	31 32 33 34 35 36 37 38

9. Circle teeth which you expect,
from your examination of the
radiographs, to have calculus on
oral or facial surfaces.

18 17 16 15 14 13 12 11	21 22 23 24 25 26 27 28
48 47 46 45 44 43 42 41	31 32 33 34 35 36 37 38

Instructor's signature: _____

Oral Epidemiology–Caries

Instruction Sheets

V-1: Basic concepts in oral epidemiology

V-2: How to use the DMFS Index

V-3: Discussion of the DMFS exercise

V-4: Caries prevention

V-5: Role of epidemiological data in public health

Exercise and Data Sheet

V-2: DMFS Index

Results Sheet

V-2: DMFS Index

Material

Student: mirror, explorer, personal radiographic survey (you will also need patience, and perhaps a computer!).

Instructor: x-ray viewboxes

Program

1. Discussion of results from Exercise IV

2. Introduction to today's topic

3. Exercises

Basic Concepts in Oral Epidemiology

Morbidity

Synonyms: disease frequency, disease dissemination, rate of disease.

The term *morbidity* is used to describe the percentage of a population which is suffering at a given point in time from a disease, for example, circulatory disturbance, eye disease, oral carcinoma, dental caries or periodontal disease. The term merely indicates whether or not the individuals have the disease. It doesn't give information about the severity, intensity, spread, extent or consequences of a disease process (e. g., are one or 30 papillae in one dentition inflamed? Are smooth surface carious lesions small or large?)

In civilized countries, the morbidity of dental caries or periodontitis is 95 to 100%. For this reason, when one must compare various civilized populations, determination of morbidity is not particularly meaningful.

Prevalence

In the field of oral epidemiology, the term *prevalence* is sometimes used in a manner similar to morbidity. But prevalence usually indicates number of diseased entities per dentition in a population. In the case of caries, it expresses the total number of carious lesions experienced during the entire lifetime, up until the time of examination (the so-called "lifetime caries experience"). See the example in Figure V-1.

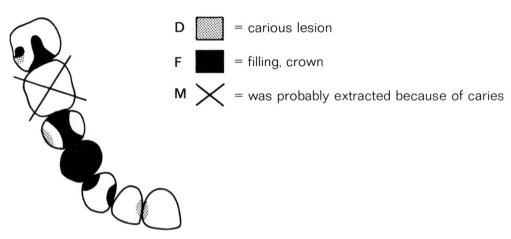

D ▨ = carious lesion

F ■ = filling, crown

M ✕ = was probably extracted because of caries

Fig. V-1

The DMF Index

D = decayed (carious)
M = missing
F = filled
T = tooth
S = surface

The DMF*T* Index expresses the sum of decayed (D), missing (M) and filled (F) *teeth* (T) per person. The DMF*S* Index scores the DMF tooth *surfaces* (S). The maximum possible DMFT score is 32, if the third molars are included, which is usually done, and 28 if these molars are not included. 32 is the maximum number of teeth which are capable of becoming carious (teeth "at risk"). In studies with adults, it is most important to note whether the third molars have been included or not.

Example of a DMFT calculation

(compare Fig. V-1)
In the quadrant depicted in the Figure, the DMFT score is 7. This number is derived as follows:

$$D = 2$$
$$F = 2$$
$$D + F = 2$$
$$M = 1$$

If one tooth has both D and F (teeth 47 and 45 in our example), then the D + F tooth is counted with the D teeth. Even better, as we have done above, a separate D + F category may be employed. In this way, the D + F can be counted as D's or as F's, depending upon the exact question one wants to answer.

The DMF Index is an index for *permanent* teeth. In the primary dentition, the comparable index is called def (e = exfoliated, lost). Since certain tooth surfaces only very seldom become carious, it has been proposed that these surfaces not even be considered when performing statistical caries studies. Only the frequently carious predilection sites are evaluated: fissures, pits, certain smooth and proximal surfaces. Occasionally, only half of the mouth is examined (partial recording).

The DMF score depends to a great extent upon how the D is judged. According to recommendations of the World Health Organization, DMFT Indices compiled for epidemiological purposes (prevalence studies) should consider only carious defects (cavities) as D, and not initial lesions (chalky spots, stained fissures).

The DMF Index cannot be a precise measurement of caries prevalence. Instead, it is only an educated estimate. The DMF score is also influenced by certain factors which have nothing to do with caries. For example, it could reflect tooth loss as a result of ortho-dontic treatment or due to periodontal disease (see graph on page 76).

The 4 primary causes of tooth loss in various age groups[1]

Epidemiological study of the Swedish population.

17,595 subjects. 34,456 extracted teeth.

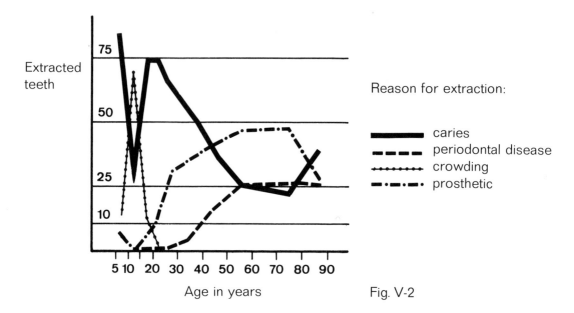

Extracted teeth

Reason for extraction:

—— caries
– – – periodontal disease
········ crowding
–·–·–· prosthetic

Age in years   Fig. V-2

[1] Lundqvist, C.: Acta Odont. Scand. 25, 289; 1967.

The DMFS Index

When this index is used, involved tooth *surfaces* (S) are counted instead of involved teeth (T).

The maximum DMFS score, when the third molars are disregarded, is 128:

4 x 2 molars with 5 surfaces each	= 40
4 x 2 bicuspids with 5 surfaces each	= 40
4 x 1 cuspid with 4 surfaces each	= 16
4 x 2 incisors with 4 surfaces each	= 32
total	= 128

Differences of opinion exist with regard to how many surface entities should be counted for molars and premolars which are crowned or lost due to caries. Usually, not all tooth surfaces were carious before a tooth was crowned or extracted. Depending upon which author you choose to follow, crowned or extracted premolars and molars are counted as 3 to 5 "F" (filled) or 3 to 5 "M" (missing) surfaces, respectively (see Instruction Sheet V-2).

A properly executed statistical study should explain clearly the maximum number of at risk tooth surfaces considered and what weight was given to crowned and extracted teeth of various tooth types.

In our example (Fig. V-1), the DMFS in the quadrant illustrated is 21 (for the total dentition it could be estimated to be 4 x 21 = 84).

$$D = 3 \quad \text{(teeth 45, 42 and 41)}$$
$$M = 5 \quad \text{(tooth 46)}$$
$$F = 12 \text{ (teeth 47, 45, 44 and 43)}$$
$$D + F = 1 \quad \text{(tooth 47)}$$

An average DMF count for an experimental group does not reveal very much to the investigator, unless the following additional information is available:

1. age
2. T or S at risk
3. definition of M for extractions and of F for crowned teeth
4. definition of D (chalky spot or frank defect?)
5. experimental conditions – field study, or were examinations done in a dental clinic?
6. combination of clinical findings with radiographic evidence of caries.

The DMF Index was originally a purely clinical index for field studies. Today, in caries prevalence studies the clinical findings are augmented by consideration of radiographs revealing the proximal carious involvement, especially when the DMFS Index is employed.

Incidence

Incidence means the *increase*, or increment, of involved entities during a selected period of observation. Incidence is a longitudinal finding and requires an initial value and a final value. Clinical incidence studies are often conducted to determine the effectiveness of agents for the inhibition of caries, dental calculus or gingivitis. Over a 2 to 3-year period, one observes the incidence in an experimental group and in a placebo or control group, the latter being identical in make-up to the experimental group.

High incidence occurs with high caries activity, but high prevalence does not necessarily indicate high caries activity. It is possible that at the time when the prevalence finding is recorded, no caries activity exists. A high prevalence value can be due to a high caries activity which was in evidence years earlier.

Caries activity is indeed dependent upon the factors which attack the tooth (plaque, carbohydrates). On the other hand, caries resistance or caries susceptibility are characteristics of the tooth itself (host). This is all relative.

Examples:

Despite high caries activity (no oral hygiene, frequent intake of carbohydrates), the caries incidence can be low, e. g., as a result of very high fluoride content of the dental enamel and of dental plaque.

Despite relatively low caries activity (relatively good oral hygiene), the caries incidence can be high, e. g., as a result of low fluoride concentration in enamel and plaque, which causes increased caries susceptibility.

DMF increments are not caused only by caries. The dentist, too, may increase the DMF, especially the DMFS, for example when he decides, for preventive reasons, to include the still caries-free buccal pit of a lower first molar into the filling he is placing in the occlusal surface of this tooth. In this way he increases the F from 1 to 2. The treatment philosophy of a school can thus influence the DMF.

How to use the DMFS Index

We determine the DMFS Index under the following conditions:

1. Third molars are not included.

2. Maximum number of at risk surfaces = 128.

3. The determination is made first on all surfaces clinically, using mirror and explorer, independent of radiographs. Subsequently, only the proximal surfaces are examined for caries radiographically, without reference to the previously obtained clinical data. Only now is the examiner ready to enter the final values into a prepared data sheet. This is done by combining and cross-checking clinical and radiographic findings. Finally, the DMFS can be calculated.

4. "D" (decayed)

Initial lesions (chalky spots – be sure to dry the teeth thoroughly!) as well as frank carious defects are counted. Be sure to examine carefully the cervical portion of the tooth crown for white spots.

Definition of grade of lesion severity

Fissures, pits

Grade 0: Healthy

Grade 1: Thin, light line. Chalky margin of fissure or pit

Grade 2: Thin, brown-to-black line

Grade 3: Frank defect, less than 2 mm in extent

Grade 4: Frank defect, greater than 2 mm

Smooth surfaces, proximal surfaces

Grade 0: Healthy

Grade 1: Chalky spot less than 2 mm in extent

Grade 2: Chalky spot greater than 2 mm

Grade 3: Frank defect less than 2 mm

Grade 4: Frank defect greater than 2 mm

A DMFS Index in which initial lesions are also included is referred to as a $D_{1-4}MFS$ Index. In the $D_{3,4}MFS$ Index, only actual carious defects or cavities are counted.

If both a smooth surface lesion of severity Grade 2 *and* a pit lesion of severity Grade 3 are detected on the *same* surface, only the more severe of the two is counted.

If no caries can be detected by clinical examination of a tooth surface, this surface is scored as healthy, even if the examiner is not certain that it really *is* healthy. Such is often the case with proximal tooth surfaces.

Definition of radiographic grade of lesion severity on proximal surfaces

Grade 1: Radiolucency in the outermost half of the enamel. Initial lesion.

Grade 2: Radiolucency also in the inner half of the enamel. No dentinal alterations.

Grade 3: Radiolucency extending completely through the enamel, with evident radio-lucency in the peripheral dentin substance.

Grade 4: Obvious dentinal radiolucency, even close to the pulp.

When radiographically detectable radiolucencies exist in fissures, pits or on smooth surfaces, one is always dealing with clinical Grade 4 carious defects, i. e., with a large cavity.

"F" (filled, = 5)

If a filling with "secondary caries" is detected on a tooth surface, that surface is counted as a "D" and not as an "F." Alternatively, a special category, "D + F," may be employed.

Gold crown or post-crown

on molars: all 5 surfaces are counted

on bicuspids: only 3 surfaces are counted

on anterior teeth: all 4 surfaces are counted

"M" (missing, = 6)

Here the same rules as those given for crowned teeth are applicable.

Practical recording of the DMFS Index

1. Clinical DMFS

It is important to proceed systematically. Use the air syringe to remove oral fluid from the teeth. Begin in the right maxillary quadrant, examining first the second molar tooth, then the first molar, and on around the arch to the central incisor. Then examine the right mandibular quadrant, again beginning with the second molar, then the first molar, and on to the incisors. Next examine the left side of the mouth, first the maxillary and then the mandibular teeth.

On each tooth, the following order of surfaces should be observed during examination: oral-occlusal-facial-distal-mesial.

Examine the teeth primarily by using your sense of sight. The explorer should be used whenever you experience doubt about a tooth surface. Dictate your findings to a classmate. He knows on which surface of which tooth you have begun the examination, and he will enter your dictated values into a prepared data collection sheet.

It is better to dictate *numbers* rather than letters of the alphabet.

0   : Zero means healthy

1, 2, 3, 4: These numbers signify decay ("D"), and express the severity of the carious lesion ($3 = D_3$).

5   : means "F" (think of filled, five, filling)

6   : means "M" (missing, extracted; "ex" = "six")

7   : means unerupted.

Example: see Fig. V-3

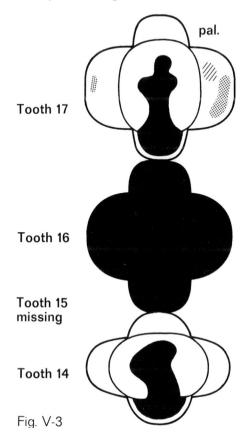

Tooth 17

Tooth 16

Tooth 15 missing

Tooth 14

Fig. V-3

Second molar, maxillary right (17)

palatal: 5 mm long chalky spot and carious defect in pit (< 2 mm). SCORE = 3

occlusal: Filling. SCORE = 5

buccal: Chalky spot, vertical extent 2 mm. SCORE = 1

distal: Healthy. SCORE = 0

mesial: Filling. SCORE = 5

Dictate: "3, 5, 1, 0, 5"

First molar, maxillary right (16)

This tooth is completely restored; i.e., all 5 of its surfaces are crowned.

Dictate: "5, 5, 5, 5, 5" (It is assumed that all five surfaces were carious prior to tooth preparation to receive the crown.)

(explanation continued on p. 82)

Second bicuspid, maxillary right (15)

This tooth, i.e., all 5 of its surfaces, had to be removed at some earlier time due to caries. The space subsequently closed.

Dictate: "6, 6, 6, 6, 6"

First bicuspid, maxillary right (14)

The mesial and occlusal surfaces are filled (mesiocclusal restoration).

Dictate: "0, 5, 0, 0, 5"

When the examination procedure described above is employed, it is really not necessary to enter the findings into a prepared data collection sheet. Continuous rows and columns of numbers are just as comprehensible, e. g.,

```
3   5   1   0   5
5   5   5   5   5
6   6   6   6   6
0   5   0   0   5    etc.
```

These same rows are then made for the other three quadrants.

Since the clinical findings will subsequently be compared with the radiographic findings, the use of a prepared data collection sheet is somewhat less abstract for the beginner. The findings shown above would look like this when entered:

	tooth 17	16	15	14
buccal	1	5	6	0
distal occlusal mesial	0 | 5 | 5	5 | 5 | 5	6 | 6 | 6	0 | 5 | 5
palatal	3	5	6	0

2. Radiographic DMFS findings

The radiographic "eye" can see proximal caries better than the clinical eye, but is not very reliable with regard to occlusal and orofacial carious lesions. For this reason, the radiographic findings serve to clarify clinical findings only in the proximal areas. (In the prepared data collection sheet, spaces for the orofacial and occlusal surfaces are not used; see below.)

Sometimes the proximal surfaces cannot be adequately examined because of overlapping caused either by the angle of x-ray projection or by the malalignment of teeth. In these instances, an "X" is entered. Thus, as far as such "X'd" proximal surfaces are concerned, the final DMFS Index is derived only from the clinical examination.

Example (see Fig. V-4, below)

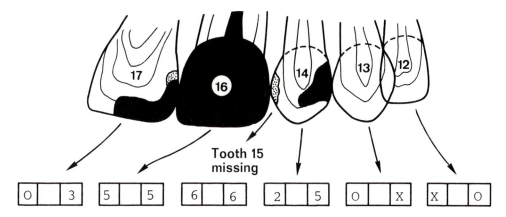

Commentary on scoring of radiographs

Tooth 17: a "3," not a "5" (filling), is entered for the mesial surface, because secondary caries with expansion into dentin (Grade 3) is noted beneath the shoulder of the filling.

Tooth 16: crowned distal and mesial surfaces: enter 5, 5.

Tooth 15: missing, was extracted because of caries. Enter 6, 6.

Tooth 14: Proximal caries distally (not detected clinically!) Enter 2, 5.

Teeth 13   Due to overlapping, two proximal surfaces cannot be adequately examined.
and 12:   Therefore, for tooth 13 enter O, X, and for tooth 12 enter X, O.

Definition of caries intensity

Caries intensity is the percentage of DMFT or, better, of DMFS entities within the teeth at risk (28) or surfaces at risk (128). The caries intensity can be expressed with or without consideration of initial lesions.

DMFS Index

Subject: _____

Examiner: _____

Date: _____

First of all, make separate clinical and radiographic diagnoses. *Do not* peek at the radiographs before you are finished with your clinical examination! Initially examine only the right side of the mouth, so that if time runs short, each student will have completed at least a "half DMFS." When filling out the prepared data collection sheet, enter only numbers. Use Exercise and Data Sheet V-2 (page 85) for entering both your clinical and radiographic findings. For radiographic findings, enter only data concerning proximal surfaces. When all data have been entered, you may compare the clinical with the radiographic figures with respect to the proximal surfaces. Determine a definitive combination finding. How well do the two compare?

Definitive Combination Finding

These data are not entered on Sheet V-2. Instead, make rows, as shown in Instruction Sheet V-2 (page 82).

Maxillary right	Mandibular left	Maxillary left	Mandibular right
_____	_____	_____	_____
_____	_____	_____	_____
_____	_____	_____	_____
_____	_____	_____	_____
_____	_____	_____	_____
_____	_____	_____	_____
_____	_____	_____	_____
_____	_____	_____	_____
_____	_____	_____	_____
_____	_____	_____	_____

DMFS Index

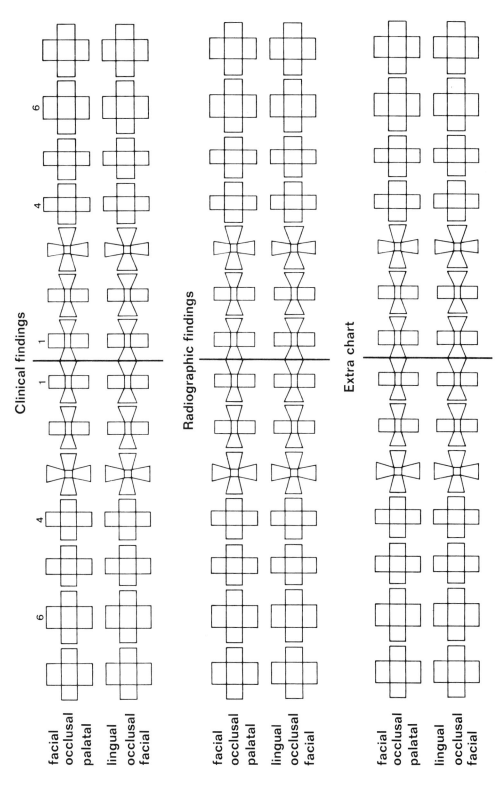

Clinical findings

Radiographic findings

Extra chart

facial
occlusal
palatal

lingual
occlusal
facial

Questions

1. On which proximal surfaces is there a discrepancy between the clinical and the radiographic findings?   _____

2. How large is the $D_{1-4}MFS$ Index?

   D surfaces (all grades)   _____
   M surfaces   _____
   F surfaces   _____
   D+F surfaces   _____   total _____

3. How large is the $D_{1-4}MFS$ Index?

   left side   _____
   right side   _____

4. How large is the $D_{3,4}MFS$ Index?

   D surfaces (only grades 3, 4) _____
   M surfaces   _____
   F surfaces   _____
   D+F surfaces   _____   total _____

5. What is the caries intensity when initial lesions are considered? Calculate it by the following formula:

$$\frac{D_{1-4}MFS \times 100}{\text{surfaces at risk}} \quad = \quad \underline{\hspace{2cm}}\%$$

6. How high is the caries intensity when initial lesions are *not* considered?

$$\frac{D_{3-4}MFS \times 100}{\text{surfaces at risk}} \quad = \quad \underline{\hspace{2cm}}\%$$

7. Calculate the DMFT from these DMFS results:

   $D_{1-4}MFT$ =   _____
   $D_{3,4}MFT$ =   _____

8. By what factor must the $D_{1-4}MFT$ value be multiplied to change it to the $D_{1-4}MFS$ value?

$$x \quad = \quad \frac{D_{1-4}MFS}{D_{1-4}MFT} \quad =$$

9. What percent must be subtracted from the $D_{1-4}MFS$ value in order to change it into the $D_{1-4}MFT$ value?

$$x\% \quad = \quad 100 \quad - \quad \frac{100 \times DMFT}{DMFS} \quad =$$

10. How high is the "Performed Treatment Index"* (number of teeth restored)?
The $D_{3,4}MFS$ may be used as a basis.

$$\frac{F \times 100}{DMFS} \quad =$$

11. How high is the necessity for treatment ("Required Treatment Index")*?
The $D_{3,4}MFS$ may be used as a basis.

$$\frac{D \times 100}{DMFS} \quad =$$

Instructor's signature: _____

* These two terms are introduced here for the first time, and are used to compare the amount of treatment with the need for treatment in a population.

DMFS Index

The results presented here are taken from a study of 27 subjects, ranging in age from 22 to 31 years. They represent epidemiological findings on caries which were compiled during the Summer semester, 1972, at the Dental Institute, University of Zurich.

1. In the entire group, 112 discrepancies were discovered between clinical and radiological findings on proximal tooth surfaces, i. e., 4.2 ± 3.0 proximal surface discrepancies per subject (range = 0 to 11).

2. $D_{1-4}MFS$ Index   range

$D_{1-4}S$	=	10.9 ± 6.9	$2 - 17$
MS	=	7.7 ± 7.8	$0 - 20$
FS	=	32.3 ± 15.7	$9 - 65$
DF + FS	=	2.5 ± 2.3	$1 - 8$
$D_{1-4}MFS$	=	53.3 ± 13.7	$30 - 80$

3. Symmetry

   $D_{1-4}MFS$ left = 25.6 ± 7.3 $11 - 40$
   right = 26.8 ± 8.0 $16 - 47$

4. $D_{3,4}MFS$ Index

$D_{3,4}S$	=	2.3 ± 1.9	$0 - 6$	Not representative of the entire
MS	=	7.7 ± 7.8	$0 - 20$	population of Switzerland
FS	=	32.1 ± 15.9	$9 - 65$	
DS + FS	=	1.4 ± 1.7	$0 - 6$	
$D_{3,4}MFS$	=	43.8 ± 15.3	$28 - 77$	Compare with Swedish students and military recruits from Finland! (see p. 90).

5. Caries intensity when chalky spots are included

   $42.0 \pm 11.0\%$ $(32 - 63\%)$

6. Caries intensity when chalky spots are not included

   $34.4 \pm 11.8\%$ $(2 - 59\%)$ This is more realistic!

7. Calculation of the DMFT from the DMFS-data

$D_{1-4}MFT$	19.1 ± 4.3	range $9 - 26$
$D_{3,4}MFT$	17.1 ± 5.1	range $3 - 25$

8. Transformation of DMFT value into DMFS

   $D_{1-4}MFT \times \underline{2.8} = D_{1-4}MFS$

9. Transformation of surface scores into tooth scores

   $D_{1-4}MFS - [D_{1-4}MFS \times 0.62] = D_{1-4}MFT$

10. Performed Treatment Index* 71.4 ± 21.4% (range = 32 – 100%)

11. Required Treatment Index*   6.4 ± 5.3% (range = 0 – 20%)

---

* See Instruction Sheet V-5.

Discussion of the DMFS Exercise

Prevalence

Let us compare the results obtained in the study performed at the University of Zurich in the Summer of 1972 with two other studies, one involving Swedish students[1], and the other Finnish recruits[2].

Comparison of the dental condition of dental students, aged 22–23 years, in 1948 and 1968.

	1948	1968	$P<$
M teeth**	1.84*	0.52	0.01
D surfaces, DS	6.38	3.32	0.01
F surfaces, FS	18.66	19.56	0.05
DMF surfaces	28.72	23.92 !	0.05
Root canals treated	1.70	0.76	
Overhanging fillings	2.74	1.28	0.01
Secondary caries	1.64	1.14	0.01
Proximal surfaces with			
periodontal defects	8.03 !	2.22 !	0.01

* N total 100, ** without third molars

The University of Zurich results are not at all comparable to the Swedish ones because from the Swedish publication we determine that the radiographic data were compiled from only 56 surfaces at risk, compared to 128 in the Zurich study!

In contrast, the study with Finnish recruits was conducted using methods similar to those presented here.

Dental condition of 154 Finnish recruits (Zurich results in parentheses)

$D_{3,4}$MFS	39.4	(43.8)
DS	17.8 !	(2.3)
FS	15.4	(32.1)
MS	6.2	(7.7)

Additional and comparable material may be reviewed in: Roth, D. G., Gier, R. E. and Warner, B. W.: The oral and physical health of students entering dental school. JADA 86, 1296–3000; 1973.

[1] Swed. dent. J. 63, 919; 1970.
[2] Finn. dent. J. 66, 301; 1970.

It is readily apparent that the amount of dental treatment which had been obtained by the Finnish recruits was less than that given to the Swiss students. The Finnish recruits had almost 7 times as many untreated carious lesions (17.8 vs 2.3 $D_{3,4}$MFS).

The most comprehensive statistical study of caries presently available is one conducted under the auspices of the United States Public Health Service[1]. The investigations were performed between 1960–1962 and the data were compiled on the basis of clinical examinations only. 6,672 subjects, aged 18 to 79 years, from 42 randomly-selected cities, were examined. Only carious defects ($D_{3,4}$) were scored. A sample from this study is reproduced in the table below, together with the results from a 1971 Swiss study.

Average caries incidence (DMFT) in 42 American cities (Caucasian race, m = male, f = female).

| Age | | Scores | | | | % Edendulous | |
		D	M	F	DMF	Max. & Mand.	Max. & Mand.
18–24	m	2.1	5.0	7.2	14.4 !	2	1
	w	1.9	5.5	7.7	15.1	1	2
35–44	m	1.2	10.0	8.1	19.3	7	7
	w	1.0	11.5	8.3	20.8	10	11
65–74	m	0.4	24.5	2.1	26.9	18	46
	w	0.3	24.8	2.8	27.9	17	53
Swiss study 1971		0.65	1.05	15.9	17.6		

These important points are noteworthy:

1. 18 to 24-year-old Americans have already lost 5.0 to 5.5 teeth.

2. In the age group 35–44 years, this figure is twice as high, as reflected also in the percent edentulousness in the table above.

3. By comparing the 1971 Swiss data with the 18 to 24-year-old age American group, one can readily see that dental students represent a select, privileged group. Although the DMF values are similar (17.6 vs 14.4/15.1), the young, white American exhibits 5 times more extracted teeth (M) and his dental treatment with fillings is only half as large (7.2/7.7 vs 15.9).

[1] National Center for Health Statistics. 1965a. Selected Dental Findings in Adults by Age, Race and Sex, United States 1960–1962. Public Health Service Publication No. 1000, Series 11, No. 7, Washington, D.C.

The American figures came from cities. Estimations in the year 1960 for the American population as a whole (180 million) were as follows:

Untreated large carious tooth surfaces ($D_{3,4}$): 3.9 per person.
Total edentulousness*: 13% of the total population.

The following table compares the total edentulousness in various age groups and in both sexes in the U.S.A. with that of Iceland[1].

Percentage of totally edentulous persons in the U.S.A. and Iceland

Age	U.S.A. (Caucasian)		Iceland	
	male	female	male	female
35 – 44	6.6	10.6	19.1	37.4
45 – 54	21.7	20.8	35.9	72.0
55 – 64	36.8	39.1	40.7	84.4

It is noteworthy that, according to the same statistical study:

22% of the population had never visited a dentist and
55% of the population went to the dentist seeking relief from pain only.

The futility of reparative dentistry

Because socioeconomic conditions are relatively similar in Switzerland and in the United States, we can transpose the figures from the American studies and get a pretty good idea about the situation in Switzerland with respect to reparative dentistry.

Assume that the task is to repair 3.9 carious tooth surfaces per person. Switzerland's population is 6 million, therefore we are dealing with 23.4 million "holes to fill." If all the dentists in Switzerland were available to work on this massive task (about 2,500 active practitioners), it is apparent that each dentist would have set before him 9,360 carious lesions which require treatment. On the average, it takes a quarter of an hour per *surface* (!) to restore a tooth, therefore it would take 2,340 hours to perform the task at hand. After one entire year of hard work (250 seven-hour working days per year) each dentist would still have 2,360 carious lesions waiting for treatment. In addition, new cavities would have formed during the year, and some old restorations would be in need of replacement. Not a single prosthesis would have been made. Furthermore, periodontal disease would have remained completely untreated.

These simple quantitative observations demonstrate that the dental problem cannot be solved through therapy alone.

---

* see also: Adult dental health in England and Wales 1968. Brit. dent. J. 129, 107; 1970.
[1] Arch. Oral Biol. 13, 571; 1968.

Caries incidence in adolescents

The caries incidence in 12 to 15-year-olds in various geographic regions of the world maybe observed in Figure V-5. It is obvious that geographic differences exist with respect to the extent of prevalence; but these may be at least partially due to methods of study and diagnostic differences.

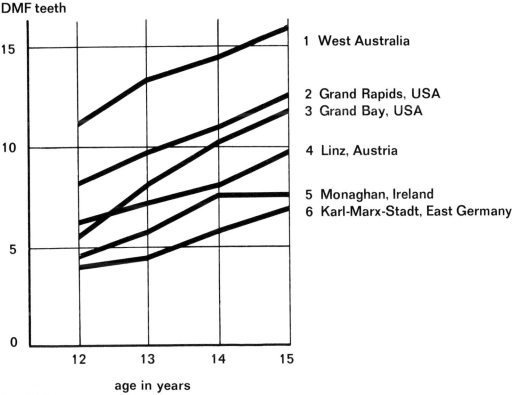

DMF teeth

1 **West Australia**

2 **Grand Rapids, USA**
3 **Grand Bay, USA**

4 **Linz, Austria**

5 **Monaghan, Ireland**
6 **Karl-Marx-Stadt, East Germany**

age in years

Fig. V-5

Caries incidence (DMFT) in Grand Rapids (Arnold 1953), Karl-Marx-Stadt (Kunzel 1969), Linz (Volk 1958), Ireland (Medical Council of Ireland 1965), Silver Bay, USA (Jordan 1964), West Australia (Halikis 1962).

Caries in Primary-Teeth

The table below provides information about the average number of def teeth per child in several highly civilized regions.

Caries incidence in primary teeth (def-T)

Years	3	4	5	6	7
Hertford (U.S.A.)	2.0	3.5	4.2	5.4	–
Providence (U.S.A.)	–	3.8	5.0	5.2	4.9
Denmark	3.5	5.2	5.7	7.2	–
Iceland	5.2	6.7	7.0	7.8	7.7
Eriswil, Rickenbach (Switzerland)	–	–	–	9.7	8.0

An article[1] published in 1970 dealing with caries in the primary teeth of 384 three-year-old children in Copenhagen, reports an average def-T of 5.4; and a def-S of 8.5!

Caries Susceptibility

Because of their various shapes and their different locations in the oral cavity, not all teeth are equally susceptible to caries. Caries susceptibility was examined[2] in 154 Finnish recruits, and the relative degrees of caries susceptibility of the various tooth types were established. This is shown below, in *increasing* order of susceptibility:

Least susceptible
1) mandibular lateral incisors
2) mandibular cuspids
3) mandibular central incisors
4) maxillary cuspids
5) mandibular first bicuspids
6) maxillary lateral incisors
7) maxillary central incisors

8) maxillary first bicuspids
9) mandibular second bicuspids
10) maxillary second bicuspids
11) maxillary second molars
12) mandibular second molars
13) maxillary first molars
Most susceptible
14) mandibular first molars

It is thus not so remarkable that the mandibular cuspids often become the "last Mohicans" of the oral cavity, to the joy of "last resort" bridge builders!

[1] Norske Tannlaegeforen. Tid. 80, 141; 1970.
[2] Finn. dent. J. 66, 301; 1970.
See also: Proc. Finn. Dent. Soc. 68, 272; 1972. Brit. Dent. J. 130, 271; 1971. Scand. J. Dent. Res. 80, 94; 1972.

The frequency distribution of the lesions among the various predilection sites is dependent upon the different susceptibilities of these sites. This refers to the order of susceptibility on page 94. These susceptibilities in turn are related to the location of the sites within the dental arch (or the oral cavity).

Percentage carious involvement of fissures and pits, proximal surfaces and smooth surfaces of selected tooth types in 13 to 20-year-olds.

	Fissures Pits	Proximal Mesial	Distal	Smooth Surfaces
Max. central incisors	3.8	43	50	0.8
Max. lateral incisors	12.4 (!)	52	40	2.4
Max. first molars	82	84	73	6.8
Mand. first molars	91	84	87	20.4
Mand. first bicuspids	10	18	49 (!)	2.8

In a study of 4,416 schoolchildren, the distribution of clinically detectable carious lesions was as follows:

Occlusal lesions   43%
Proximal lesions   31%
Buccal-lingual lesions 26%

In the 30 to 35-year age group, the percentage of proximal lesions is higher.

Amalgam Fanatic:

A dental professor said: "Really, a
Hole-filling technique's so silly, a
Dentist these days
Who still does it that way's
Possessed by amalgamophilia"!

Incidence and Increment

How rapidly do new carious defects occur?

The caries incidence can be estimated from prevalence studies of various age groups. But more precise information can only be obtained from longitudinal studies, in which the increase in caries in the same group is measured continuously. Marthaler[1] observed a group of Zurich school children over a 7-year period. These children did not receive any special type of caries preventive measures.

Caries incidence in Zurich children from 1958 to 1965

| | DMFS | | DMFS Increment |
	7-year-olds	14-year-olds	per year
all lesions $(D_{1-4}MFS)$ without consideration of early lesions	6.7	44.7	5.4
$(D_{3,4}MFS)$	3.1	27.5	3.5

Intensity of Caries

If we assume 128 surfaces at risk in the above study, the 14-year-olds already had 44.7 carious surfaces; that's 35% of all surfaces. Fortunately, in the interim the situation in the Canton of Zurich has improved considerably, thanks to the "Caries Prevention Program."

Additional recommended literature

Berman, D. S., Slack, G. L.: Dental caries in English school children. Brit. dent. J. 133, 529; 1972.

Marthaler, T. M.: A standardized system of recording dental conditions. Helv. Odont. Acta 10, 1–18; 1966.

Marthaler, T. M.; Epidemiologie von Zahnkaries, Gingivitis und Zahnstein bei 7646 Schweizer Schulkindern. Schweiz. Mschr. Zahnheilk. 78, 19; 1968.

Möller, I. J. and S. Poulsen: A standardized system for diagnosing, recording and analyzing dental caries data. Scand. J. dent. Res. 81, 1–11; 1973.

Murray, J. J.: Adult dental health in fluoride and non-fluoride areas. Brit. dent. J. 131, 487; 1971.

Samuelson, G., Grahnen, H., Lindström, G.: An epidemiological study of child health and nutrition ina northern Swedish county. Odont Revy 22, 189; 1971.

Van Erp, N.A.K.M., Meyer-Jansen, A. C.: A caries study of the temporary molars and its significance for their conservative care. Netherlands Dent. J., Suppl. 5, 77; 1970.

[1] Marthaler, T. M.: Schweiz. Mschr. Zahnheilk. 78, 134; 1968.

Caries Prevention

Marthaler[1] reported the caries incidence in 5,819 school children in 16 Zurich districts in the years 1964 and 1968. In these districts, the children brushed their teeth under supervision 6 times per year with a fluoride-containing solution, and were provided with oral hygiene information. The following figures derive not from an incidence study on the same children in 1964 and 1968, but rather from two caries prevalence studies on the school children in these 2 years.

Incidence of caries ($D_{3,4}$MFS) in Zurich districts in the years 1964 and 1968. Numbers of children examined are in parentheses.

	10-year-olds	12-year-olds
1964	9.52 (487)	17.14 (473)
1968	6.14 (660)	11.56 (639)
Reduction	36%	33%

The caries reduction is even more striking when anterior teeth alone are considered.

Caries incidence among anterior teeth ($D_{3,4}$MFS) in Zurich districts in 1963 and 1967.

	10-year-olds	12-year-olds
1963	1.25	2.57
1967	0.28	0.87
Reduction	78%	66%

It is interesting that very great differences exist among the various districts in Switzerland, and even within the Canton of Zurich itself. A summary of the results compiled by the Zurich Experimental Caries Research Laboratory[2] in 40 districts on a total of 7,046 children brings this out very well.

Average caries incidence ($D_{3,4}$MFS) in 10 to 15-year-olds in 40 Swiss districts

All 40 districts	24.5
Küsnacht (Canton of Zurich)	13.2
Ossingen (Canton of Zurich)	24.5
Flumenthal (Canton of Solothurn)	36.7

[1] Marthaler, T.: Helv. odont. Acta 16, 45; 1972.

[2] Macciachini, G.: Kariesprophylaxe und zahnärztlicher Sanierungszustand. Schweiz. Mschr. Zahnheilk. 80, 1235; 1970.

In the data cited, the caries incidence was expressed using the $D_{3,4}MFS$. Other authors use the $D_{3,4}MFT$, or the $D_{1-4}MFT$ and $D_{1-4}MFS$. In order to render these data comparable, the reciprocal relationships of these different methods of expressing results should be known.

a) The DMF-Surface index is approximately twice as large as the DMF-Tooth index (see, for example, Gulzow et al.[1]).

b) After eruption of the second molars, the DMFS index is about 1.5 times larger than the $D_{3,4}MFS$ index, if clinical and radiographic early lesions are included.

c) The $D_{3,4}MFS$ is about two-thirds of the $D_{1-4}MFS$.

d) It is worth remembering that after eruption of the permanent dentition the $D_{3,4}MF$-Tooth index is about 10–20% smaller than the age, in districts where no organized caries prophylaxis is performed.

For example:

12-year-olds:	12 minus 1.2 to 2.4 = 9.6 to 10.8 DMFT
14-year-olds:	14 minus 1.4 to 2.8 = 11.2 to 12.6 DMTF
recruits (age 20):	20 minus 2.0 to 4.0 = 16.0 to 18.0 DMFT

These rules of thumb are valid for the age range 10 to 20 years.

According to what we have said thus far, the following rough estimates could also be made for the 14-year-olds from the often reported $D_{3,4}MFT$ scores:

$D_{3,4}MFS$ = 2 x 11.2 to 12.6 = 22.4 to 25.2
$D_{1,4}MFS$ = 1.5 x 22.4 to 25.2 = 33.6 to 37.8

In districts where organized caries prophylaxis is performed, the $D_{3,4}MFS$ is today clearly smaller than 20. This is also seen from statistics dealing with effects of water fluoridation (Table V-4).

The statistics from Hastings show:

1. The DMFS is almost 2½ times higher than the DMFT when the caries prevalence is high (1954).

2. The DMFS is only twice as high as the DMFT where the caries prevalence is reduced (1970).

3. Caries reduction figures calculated on the basis of DMFS indices are higher than those calculated from DMFT scores.

[1] Gulzow, H. J., et al.: Schweiz. Mschr. Zahnheilk. 78, 1195; 1968.

Fluoridation of communal drinking water cannot be discussed here in detail, but Table V-4 (below) is presented as an example of the cariostatic efficacy of water fluoridation in children. The concept that the effect of water fluoridation can no longer be demonstrated as age increases is not valid[1]. For example, when Hartlepool (1.5 ppm F in the drinking water) is compared with York (0.2 ppm F in the drinking water), the prevalence of smooth surface, occlusal and pit lesions is smaller by 50%, 37% and 24%, respectively[1].

Caries epidemiology:

> "With double-blind studies," said he,
> "We get valid data, you see"?
> "With patience you'll prove
> Fluoride's right in the groove
> Ep-i-dem-i-o-log-i-cal-ly"!

Table V-4
Average DMFT and DMFS indices in 14 and 15-year-old children in Hastings (New Zealand) in 1954 and 16 years later, after introduction of drinking water fluoridation (in parentheses, number of children examined)[2]

Age				1954		1970	% Reduction
14	m	(62)	DMFT	13.9	(90)	6.1	56
			DMFS	31.3		12.1	61
	w	(66)	DMFT	14.8	(113)	7.5	49
			DMFS	36.1		14.6	60
15	m	(44)	DMFT	15.9	(77)	7.9	50
			DMFS	39.2		16.2	59
	w	(44)	DMFT	17.7	(80)	9.1	48
			DMFS	45.9		18.6	59

[1] Jackson, D., Murray, J. J., Fairpo, C. G.: Life-long benefits of fluoride in drinking water. Brit. dent. J., 134, 419; 1973.

[2] Ludwig, T. G.: Hastings fluoridation project. VI. Dental effects between 1954 and 1970. New Zealand D. J. 67, 155; 1971.

Role of Epidemiological Data in Public Health

DMF data are useful for expressing quantitatively the amount of treatment performed and the amount of dental treatment which is required within a group of children.

Performed Treatment Index = percentage of fillings in the DMF Index

$$\frac{F}{DMFT} \times 100 \quad \text{or} \quad \frac{F}{DMFS} \times 100$$

Required Treatment Index = percentage of carious defects in the DMF Index

$$\frac{D}{DMFT} \times 100 \quad \text{or} \quad \frac{D}{DMFS} \times 100$$

Walsh[1] published treatment indices for various countries:

Australia	26
U.S.A.	23
England	14
Norway	86
New Zealand	72

Such treatment indices must be very carefully interpreted, because the degree of caries prevalence is an important factor as well. It is obvious from Walsh's report that the Performed Treatment Index of New Zealand, the country with the world's most highly organized public dental service (New Zealand Dental Nurses), is not as favorable as that of Norway. The point to remember, of course, is that in New Zealand caries *prevalence* is almost twice as high as it is in Norway ($D_{3,4}$MFT for 15-year-olds in Norway is 8.0, in New Zealand 15.0). It is quite a bit simpler to provide complete treatment for the Norwegian children because they have a much smaller caries prevalence than New Zealand children.

In Switzerland, too, these differences can be quite pronounced. Figures from the Zurich Experimental Caries Research Laboratory show the Performed Treatment Index among 13 to 15-year-olds in the district of Fiesch to be 16%, in Kilchberg 80%. The Required Treatment Index in Oberrieden is only 12%, but in Fiesch it is 72%.

[1] Walsh, J.: New Zealand Dent. J. 66, 143; 1970.

Caries incidence and Performed Treatment Index in Zurich schoolchildren

85% of the children in the public schools of the city of Zurich were treated in 13 school dental clinics having a total of 43 treatment chairs. Of the 37,000 patients, 4,000 were of preschool age[1].

The number of appointments for treatment of dental caries in 1969 was 145,000; for orthodontic treatment: 27,000. Seven percent of the children wore some type of orthodontic apparatus.

Upon leaving school, between the ages of 16 and 20 years, all children receive a "birthday ticket" which entitles them to an oral examination by a private dentist, with costs paid by the State. This service is provided under terms of a government "Dental Care for Youth" program. For children from economically disadvantaged families, the State assumes 70% of all treatment costs, up to a maximum of 150 Swiss francs. In 1969, 81% of the "birthday tickets" which had been distributed were used.

Caries incidence in primary teeth

Kindergarten: (5 to 6-year-olds)

1959: 10.4% had caries-free deciduous dentitions

1969: 30.1% had caries-free deciduous dentitions

Kindergarten children from working class neighborhoods have more caries than children from "white collar" neighborhoods:

Caries-free kindergarten children in percent per school district, 1969 (diagnosis based on visual examination only):

Zurichberg	41.8
Waidberg	36.7
Uto	33.7
Letzi	29.4
Limmat	29.3
Glattal	25.9
Schwammendingen	23.4

[1] ZWR 79, 1048; 1970.

Caries in the permanent dentition

Proximal surface caries detected radiographically through the use of bite-wing films in 16-year-old Zurich school children (1st and 2nd premolars and molars).

Caries-free	1961 (N = 434)	36 percent
	1969 (N = 531)	51 percent
Filled or carious	1961	50 percent
	1969	41 percent
Extracted	1961	14 percent
	1969	8 percent

Radiographic caries incidence in proximal surfaces of 1st molars

Caries-free	1961	16 percent
	1969	36 percent
Filled or carious	1961	48 percent
	1969	47 percent
Extracted	1961	36 percent
	1969	16 percent

Treatment performed in Zurich school dental clinics, 1965 and 1969

		Deciduous teeth	Permanent teeth	Per child
Surfaces restored by silver amalgam	1965	27,126	106,724	3.9
	1969	39,146	89,550	3.5
		+ 44%	– 16%	
Surfaces restored by silicate cement	1965		13,260	
	1969		8,679	
			– 34%	

As a provider of dental service, the dentist is obligated to be at least somewhat informed regarding the extent of carious destruction in the population. The layman knows that there is "a lot of decay." But how much?

You should be aware of the following figures[1] if you are to fulfill your "public relations" role:

[1]Adapted from J. Dent. Child., February, 1970.

1. At least 96% of the population suffers from some type of dental problem.

2. Almost 50% of persons over 55 years of age have lost their natural teeth.

3. More than 50% of 2-year-old children have caries.

4. In 15-year-olds, more than half the teeth are carious.

5. Each year, almost 350 new cases of oral cancer occur in Switzerland. This type of cancer has one of the lowest survival rates among the various types of cancer.

6. Per 100 recruits, the American army must perform 500 fillings and 80 extractions, and must construct 25 bridges and 20 prostheses. During the Viet Nam experience, one out of every 12 U.S. soldiers was off duty because of dental problems, the time lost ranging from a matter of hours up to five days.

7. Experts see the necessity for dental treatment in civilized countries as being so great that it is neither reasonable nor possible to remedy this situations through treatment and replacement alone. The emphasis must be upon the prevention of dental damage before it starts. In order to achieve this goal, we will have to concentrate our energies upon the child population. The young must be brought through childhood and adolescence with healthy mouths. Only in this way can the treatment problem ever be solved.

Caries Prevention:

> Dr. Marthaler stood 'fore the class
> With toothbrush and fluoride and glass.
> He cried: "Hey, kids, it's the truth!
> We can stop holes in your tooth!
> So brush your teeth, and do it fast"!

Recommended literature

Marthaler, T. M.: Reduction of caries, gingivitis and calculus after eight years of preventive measures-Observations in seven communities. Helv. Odont. Acta 16, 69; 1972.

Turner, G.: Organization in the School Dental Service. Brit. dent. J., 131, 511; 1971.

Gingiva

Instruction Sheets

VI-1: The gingival complex
VI-2: Gingival recession
VI-3: The gingival sulcus

Exercise and Data Sheets

VI-1: Measurement of the width of the attached gingiva
VI-2: Measurement of gingival recession
VI-3: Measurement of gingival sulcus depth

Results Sheet

VI-2 and VI-3: Exercise Results

Material

Student: cotton pliers, mouth mirror, explorer
Instructor: Schiller's iodine solution, periodontal probes, millimeter strips, force meter
          (0–100 g)

Program

1. Discussion of the results from Exercise V, "Oral Epidemiology – Caries"
2. Introduction to today's topic
3. Exercises

The Gingival Complex

The gingivae may be considered to have 3 component parts:

1. The marginal gingiva, also called the gingival cuff, the free gingiva or the "M" gingival unit
2. The interdental papilla, or "P" unit
3. The attached gingiva, also called the gingiva propria, or "A" unit.

The free gingiva is separated from the stippled, keratinized, coral pink attached gingiva by the free gingival groove, which is often not clinically apparent. It is bordered facially in the maxilla, and facially and lingually in the mandible by the mucogingival junction (linea girlandiformis), which borders upon the mobile, unkeratinized alveolar mucosa. The interdental papillary gingiva is made up of a facial and an oral papilla, connected to each other through a saddle-shaped col area. The gingival sulcus is the crevice bordered by the internal surface of the folded-over gingival margin, the enamel and the beginning of the epithelial attachment (junctional epithelium). Histologically, this sulcus is about 0.5 mm deep; upon gentle probing the sulcus can be measured clinically at 0.5 to 2 mm in depth.

The transition line between the attached gingiva and the alveolar mucosa is called the mucogingival junction. This structure can be rendered distinctly visible by the application of Schiller's iodine solution[1]. Immediately the alveolar mucosa picks up the stain whereas the heavily keratinized attached gingiva stains to a slight degree only. The mucogingival border can also be located through finger palpation, on the basis of the different mobilities of the attached gingiva and the alveolar mucosa upon their underlying structures[2].

The attached gingiva is of varying width. It is physiologically narrower at the insertion of lip and cheek frena. When gingival recession occurs, the attached gingiva becomes narrower, this time on a pathological basis.

[1] Parodontologie 12, 1515; 1958.

[2] Summary of the literature: Helv. odont. Acta 15, 118; 1971.

Measurement of the Width of the Attached Gingiva

Subject: _____

Examiner: _____

Date: _____

1. Stain the alveolar mucosa and the attached gingiva orally and facially, both in maxilla and mandible around 3 teeth, using Schiller's iodine solution.

2. Where is the mucogingival junction located on the palatal? Write your answer:

3. Measure the width of the attached gingiva (A) using a graduated periodontal probe over the labial root prominence, parallel to the root. The distance to be measured is from the "most apical extent of the free gingival margin" (where the stippling begins) to the mucogingival junction. The easiest way to do this is by using the graduated probe to measure from the gingival margin to the mucogingival junction, then to subtract the depth of the gingival sulcus from this figure (see page 114). Perform this measurement also around teeth with gold crowns or post crowns (note these in the chart below). Measure over both mesiobuccal and distobuccal roots of maxillary and mandibular molars.

Enter the millimeter measurements above or below the respective tooth numbers in the chart. Cross out missing teeth. Note cast crowns.

Facial aspect of maxilla	21	22	23	24	25	26m	26d	27m	27d
Facial aspect of mandible	31	32	33	34	35	36m	36d	37m	37d
Oral aspect of mandible	31	32	33	34	35	36m	36d	37m	37d

Calculate the average width of the attached gingiva.
N = number of entities observed

$N_{max. facial}$ = _____ , $\bar{x}$ = _____

$N_{mand. facial}$ = _____ , $\bar{x}$ = _____

$N_{mand. oral}$ = _____ , $\bar{x}$ = _____

On which tooth was the smallest "A" measured? _____ How wide was it? _____

Instructor's signature: _____

Gingival Recession

If we are to understand gingival recession, we must first agree upon a few definitions. Normally, after complete eruption of a tooth, the healthy, inflammation-free gingiva covers the cervical two to three millimeters of the tooth crown like a collar. For this reason, differentiation is made between the *clinical* and the *anatomical* crown.

Clinical crown: This is the visible portion of a tooth.

Anatomical crown: The boundary of the anatomical crown is the cementoenamel junction (CEJ), which is often covered by the free gingival margin.

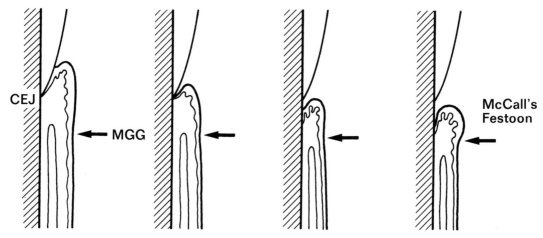

Fig. VI-1   CEJ: cementoenamel junction. MGG: mucogingival border

Throughout life, the clinical crown becomes longer as the gingiva and the periodontal bone recede (recession). In due course, the cementoenamel junction and the cervical portion of the root cementum are exposed, a process referred to as "denudation." The entire course of events has been called "passive eruption." Such recession can occur entirely in the absence of marginal inflammation, and it may occur at quite different rates in different individuals. Often, however, an existing marginal gingivitis masks the initial stages of gingival recession, because it results in gingival enlargement. Due to the exposure of the cementoenamel junction, cervical tooth sensitivity is often the first subjective symptom of recession.

Review of possible etiological factors:

Age

Gottlieb (1927) referred to recession (which he termed "retraction") as "physiological passive tooth eruption." On the other hand, there may be no recession, even in a 76-year-old!

Tooth position anomalies

In the anterior area, certain anomalies of tooth position (e. g., anterior protrusion from a narrow apical base, "labioversion") are associated with very thin buccal alveolar bone. The marginal osseous structure may even be absent; a condition then called "dehiscence." Perforation of the bone around the middle portion of the root is called "fenestration." The question becomes: Are dehiscences and fenestrations causes or consequences of recession?

Tooth movement

Tooth movement due to abnormal forces can theoretically lead to relationships similar to those just mentioned in terms of tooth position anomalies. Fortunately, this is seldom, if ever, a cause of recession.

Occlusal trauma

Stillman (1921) held occlusal trauma responsible for what he called "gingival clefts." These were narrow, crevice-like "recessions" which, if left untreated, progressed with inflammation. But recession is also found associated with teeth upon which no occlusion at all occurs, and this both in children and in adults. Furthermore, tooth mobility is never increased in cases of recession ("No occlusal trauma without increased tooth mobility," see Chapter XVI).

Buccal and lingual frena

The insertions of buccal and lingual frena do, indeed, lead to a narrowing of the attached gingiva, but in only 3% of cases are they directly involved with recession.

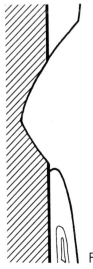

Abrasion from toothbrushing

Pronounced gingival recession is often associated with intensive horizontal "scrubbing" with the toothbrush. When such is the background, the recession will usually be observed in close proximity to wedge-shaped cervical defects (or "notches," see Fig. VI-2). Most certainly the mechanical factor of overzealous toothbrushing is the most significant cause of recession. The aging process (periodontal atrophy), of course, is another underlying cause of recession.

Fig. VI-2

The gingiva may also recede as a consequence of connective tissue shrinkage, subsequent to the treatment of periodontal pockets in patients with marginal periodontitis. Recession also occurs frequently after extraction of adjacent teeth. Again, marginal irritation (subgingival calculus, orthodontic bands, filling margins) may also cause vertical, crevice-like gingival recessions called "Stillman's clefts."

Initially, recession occurs only on the facial aspect of the root. The tips of the interdental papillae maintain their normal positions between the teeth for a long time after recession is clearly manifest.

Recession, of course, leads to narrowing of the attached gingiva. The distance from the mucogingival boundary to the free gingival margin becomes smaller. Recession is frequently seen in connection with a firm, rolled-up, fibrotic thickening of the gingival margin, and a narrowing of the attached gingiva. It is as though a wall were being established to prevent the apically progressing and destructive process from continuing further. Such marginal thickenings in the cervical area are referred to as "McCall's festoons" (see Fig. VI-1).

Literature summary in Periodontal Abstracts 17, 45–50; 1969 (June).

See also: O'Leary, T., Drake, R. B., Crump, P. P., Allen, M. F.: The incidence of recession in young males: A further study. J. Periodont. 42, 264; 1971.

Measurement of Gingival Recession

Subject: _____

Age: _____

Examiner: _____

Date: _____

Method

Using a graduated periodontal probe, measure the facial and oral gingival recession at its most pronounced point. Measure from the cementoenamel junction (CEJ) to the free gingival margin (GM). If GM lies directly at the CEJ, a recession of 2 mm is assumed and this figure is entered into the chart.

If the gingival margin lies on the root surface, 2 mm should be added to the CEJ–GM measurement.

Examples:

Fig. VI-2

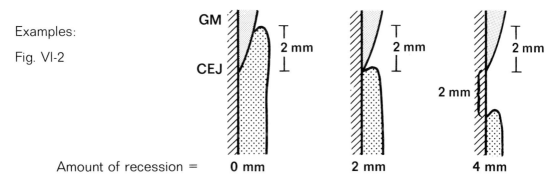

Amount of recession =   0 mm   2 mm   4 mm

It is seldom easy to locate the cementoenamel junction visually. You must use an explorer and your sense of touch. In addition, you may detect color differences between enamel (white) and root cementum (light yellow). The sensitivity of the tooth cervix may help. But be careful to avoid mistaking a pathological cervical carious chalky spot for the CEJ! If fillings are present along the cervical lines, you have no other choice but to estimate the position of the CEJ. Compare the neighboring teeth!

Often the gingival margin is so thickened that the CEJ-GM measurement exceeds 2 mm. In such cases, enter a "zero" in the chart, not a negative number.

Exercise

Choose the side of the mouth where the most recession areas are present. Only those teeth which are free of post crowns and cast crowns should be considered. In the chart (page 112), cross out teeth whereon recession cannot be measured (crowns, overlying calculus), or any which are missing.

In the case of molars, measure facially over the mesial and distal roots; orally over the palatal root.

Enter your values in the chart, above or below the tooth number. Be sure to enter "zero" values as well!

Which side of the mouth was examined?   left   right

								pal.			pal.	
Max.	Facial	1 2 3 4 5	m6		6d	m7		7d
	Oral			6p			7p	
Mand.	Oral	1 2 3 4 5	m6		6d	m7		7d
	Facial							

1. How many cervical areas (CA) were evaluated?   N = _____

2. How many CA show recession greater than 2 mm?   _____

3. How many show no recession?   _____

4. On how many CA did you find recession on the oral aspect?   _____

5. On how many CA did you find recession on the facial aspect?   _____

6. On which CA are "McCall's festoons" present?   _____

7. Calculate the average [x̄] recession (sum [Σ] of the recessions divided by the number [N] of cervical areas examined).

Maxilla

Facial: $\bar{x} = \dfrac{\Sigma}{N} = $ _____ $\bar{x} = $ _____

Palatal: $\bar{x} = \dfrac{\Sigma}{N} = $ _____ $\bar{x} = $ _____

Mandible

Facial: $\bar{x} = \dfrac{\Sigma}{N} = $ _____ $\bar{x} = $ _____

Lingual: $\bar{x} = \dfrac{\Sigma}{N} = $ _____ $\bar{x} = $ _____

Max. + Mand. $\bar{x} = \dfrac{total\ \Sigma}{total\ N} = $ _____ $\bar{x} = $ _____

Instructor's signature: _____

The Gingival Sulcus

We must differentiate between the *clinical* and the *histological* gingival sulcus. The histological gingival sulcus has a depth of about 0.5 mm. Clinically, using 20–40 Ponds of force on a graduated instrument, the sulcus may be probed to a depth of between 1 and 3 mm without causing the patient any pain. The histological sulcus can also be "blown open" with an air stream.

A pathologically deepened clinical sulcus is called a gingival pocket. It is an early sign of marginal periodontitis.

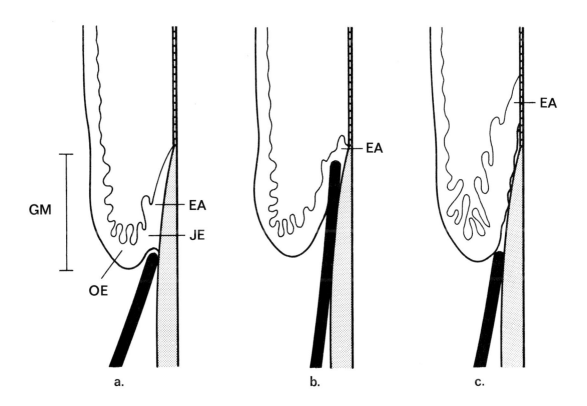

Fig. VI-3:   a. Histological sulcus,   b. Clinical sulcus with flexible plastic probe in situ, c. Pathologically deepened sulcus. Note deep proliferation of epithelium. The in vivo situation is an actual crevice. Probe at entrance of pocket. (OE = oral epithelium JE = junctional epithelium EA = epithelial attachment GM = free gingival).

Measurement of Gingival Sulcus Depth

Subject: _____

Age: _____

Examiner: _____

Date: _____

Method

Insert the graduated periodontal probe into the gingival sulcus as nearly as possible parallel to the long axis of the tooth root until you meet resistance and the patient feels mild discomfort. Don't be too gentle! Exert 20–30 Ponds of force. Check the amount of force applied using a force gauge. Interproximally, it is not possible to insert the probe exactly parallel to the long axis of the tooth; rather, the probe must be positioned on a slight diagonal toward the col area. You will frequently encounter bleeding from the gingival sulcus, but this should not influence your measurements.

Exercise

1. Measure the sulcus depth facially, orally, mesially and distally on each tooth in the maxillary quadrant which has the least amount of dental work. On the maxillary molars, measure orally only above the palatal root. Facially in the molar area, you should use the probe along both mesial and distal roots, as well as in the furcation area. Enter measurements in the chart!

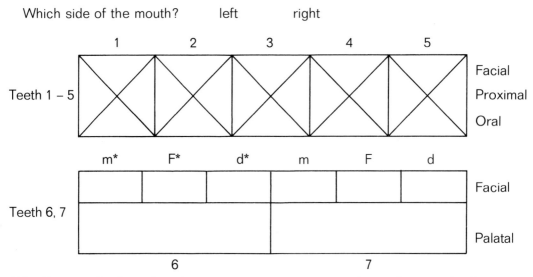

* F = Furcation (midbuccal area), m = measurement over mesial root, d = over distal root

2. What was the largest measurement? _____ mm

3. Was this measurement made in a sulcus or in a pocket?

   Sulcus [   ]   Pocket [   ]

4. Calculate the average sulcus depth

facial   N = $\bar{x}$ = _____

oral   N = $\bar{x}$ = _____

distal   N = $\bar{x}$ = _____

mesial   N = $\bar{x}$ = _____

Instructor's signature: _____

Exercise Results

1. Measurement of the width of the attached gingiva in 22 students during the summer semester, 1972:

		Range
Maxilla, facial aspect	2.8 ± 1.0 mm	0.9 – 4.7
Mandible, facial aspect	2.1 ± 0.7 mm	0.3 – 3.2
Mandible, oral aspect	2.7 ± 0.7 mm	1.5 – 3.8

A minimal width (0.0 – 0.5 mm) was found:

	tooth number
7 times at	33, 43
5 times at	34, 44
4 times at	17, 27
4 times at	31, 41

During the winter semester, 1971–72, the following measurements were obtained from 25 different students of similar age:

Maxillary facial	3.7 ± 1.0 mm
Mandibular facial	2.4 ± 0.8 mm
Mandibular oral	3.2 ± 1.0 mm

2. Measurement of gingival recession

a) Per subject, the cervical root surface was denuded in 2.7 ± 3.1 teeth (range 0–9!) per half-mouth (14 teeth).

b) Per subject, absence of any recession at all was found on only 1.9 teeth of the half-mouth (range 0–8!)

c, d) Recession was present on the facial aspect with a frequencyof 79%, whereas orally it was 57%.

e) McCall's festoons were discovered in 7 of the 22 students, most often around the cuspid tooth. Is this a defense mechanism against recession?

f) Comparing the recession data obtained from the 22 subjects in summer semester of 1972 with the figures of winter semester 1971–72, (7 teeth in the maxilla and 7 in the mandible on one side of the mouth) we see in summary:

		Summer Semester 1972	Range	Winter Semester 1972
Maxilla	facial	1.4 ± 0.8 mm	0.1 – 3.0	1.9 ± 0.5
	oral	0.8 ± 0.6 mm	0.0 – 2.0	1.4 ± 0.4
Mandible	facial	1.3 ± 0.6 mm	0.4 – 2.2	1.9 ± 0.6
	oral	1.0 ± 0.7 mm	0.4 – 2.2	1.9 ± 0.9
Maxilla & Mandible		1.1 ± 0.6 mm	0.5 – 2.4	

There are clear variations in the values for the two groups of subjects. The differences in the width of the attached gingiva as well as the amount of recession are probably not true differences, but rather are due to the error of the method.

In the literature, the following figures are given regarding the frequency of recession. Gorman[1] found recession in 62 % of 16 to 25-year-olds. O'Leary et al.[2] reported that in 592 recruits, age 19.5 years, 27.7 % exhibited denudation of the CEJ. Recession varied in different areas of the mouth:

Max. molars and bicuspids	16.1%
Mand. molars and bicuspids	6.2%
Max. anterior teeth	5.7%
Mand. anterior teeth	5.9%

The large difference in frequency of recession noted in our exercises as compared to the data from the literature appears to be due to differences in definition of the term recession.

See also Stahl and Morris[3], who present a recession index (R.I.) for the rapid performance of epidemiological investigations.

$$R.I. = \frac{\text{teeth with recession} \times 100}{\text{number of examined teeth per person}}$$

3. Measurement of sulcus depth

a) In 22 subjects, where 4 measurements were performed per tooth in one quadrant, the highest average value was 2.9 ± 0.5 mm; the highest single value was 4.0 mm.

b) The highest value in any one subject was measured in a true pocket in only 2 instances.

[1] J. Periodont. 38, 316; 1967.
[2] Periodontics 6, 109; 1968.
[3] Periodont. 26, 180; 1955.

c) The average clinical sulcus depths were:

		Range
facial	1.6 ± 0.4 mm (1.55)	1.0 – 2.2 mm
oral	1.5 ± 0.4 mm (1.50)	0.9 – 2.2 mm
distal	1.8 ± 0.5 mm (1.97)	1.0 – 2.9 mm
mesial	2.0 ± 0.5 mm (2.01)	1.2 – 2.8 mm

These figures agree well with the averages obtained from an earlier study of 20 other course participants; the averages are given in parentheses.

Gingival Recession:

> A stripper, Miss Tooth Neck by name,
> Shed her covering with no hint of shame.
> Her gingivae yielded
> To a brush wrongly wielded.
> Her sulcus depth, though, stayed the same.

Oral Hygiene

Instruction Sheets

VII-1: Determining oral cleanliness – plaque indices

VII-2: Dental calculus indices

VII-3: Plaque disclosing agents (Plaque detectors)

Exercise and Data Sheets

VII-1: Measurement of plaque

VII-2: Measurement of dental calculus

Results Sheet

VII-1: Measurement of plaque

VII-2: Discussion of exercise results

Material

Student: cotton pliers, periodontal probe, mouth mirror

Instructor: disclosing agents

Program

1. Discussion of results from Exercise VI, "Gingiva"

2. Introduction to today's topic

3. Exercises

Determining Oral Cleanliness

Synopsis

Caries and marginal periodontitis are chronic infectious diseases. The phrase "No bacteria = no caries and no inflammatory periodontal disease" emphasizes the significance of a clean, or an unclean, oral cavity. But what is a clean mouth? What is a "dirty" dentition? When does uncleanliness begin? Is it possible to get the teeth really clean with a toothbrush alone? Is it possible to motivate people toward good oral hygiene?

These questions can only be answered by employing techniques which measure or score the degree of cleanliness or uncleanliness of the oral cavity. Such techniques may be divided into those which measure microbial plaque and those which measure hard deposits (dental calculus)[1].

Measurement of soft deposits

Depending upon the question being asked in an investigation, various indices or semi-quantitative methods may be employed.

The Oral Hygiene Index (OHI) has become the index of choice for epidemiological studies of the degree of dental uncleanliness in large populations. The index is simple to use, requires little time and distinguishes between soft and hard deposits. The OHI-S (S = simplified) is even simpler; see page 123.

The Quigley-Hein Index is a relatively simple and sensitive index which is indicated for determination of the degree of plaque removal through oral hygiene measures in fairly large groups.

In plaque incidence studies, especially studies of the relationship between plaque and the marginal gingiva, the Plaque Index (PI) of Silness and Löe is most reliable. This index is often used for testing anti-plaque substances in oral preparations.

Planimetry or gravimetry of plaque are more complicated and are only used in special investigations and in small groups of subjects.

Knowledge and use of the more important calculus and plaque indices will be of extraordinary significance in the future. If government-sponsored dental insurance becomes a reality, as is being promoted in many countries, the insurance companies and the dentists can accept such a challenge only on the stipulation that the "policy holders" demonstrate their practice of adequate oral hygiene. Those people with "dirty mouths" deserve no government support for treatment made necessary because of their own

---

[1]   Short inclusive review:
   Tooth accumulated materials. A review and classification. J. Periodont. 40, 407; 1969.

laziness. In the future it will become commonplace to distinguish the "clean" from the "dirty," orally speaking! Towards this end, a quantitative, objective method is needed for periodically checking the patient's cooperation. The Oral Hygiene Index may serve this purpose. The holder of a government-sponsored dental insurance policy would receive an Oral Health Booklet, in which his degree of oral cleanliness would be entered at a yearly examination. If the patient failed to keep up his oral hygiene satisfactorily, e. g., if his OHI score exceeded 2.0, he would lose his right to government insurance funds to cover his dental treatment costs.

Plaque Indices

The Oral Hygiene Index (OHI)

The original OHI was published by Greene and Vermillion[1] in 1957, and simplified by the same authors[2] in 1964 (OHI-S, OHI-Simplified). We will not use this index in our exercises, because it is not sensitive enough for evaluation of the oral hygiene status in dental students. We will discuss it briefly, however, because many epidemiological studies employ it, and an index score without knowledge of its origins is not very valuable.

Principle

The OHI score is composed of two components: the "oral debris" value and the "dental calculus" value. The term "oral debris" signifies "plaque plus materia alba plus food remnants" (soft deposits).

The soft and hard deposits are scored on the facial and oral surfaces of six teeth. The teeth with the heaviest deposits in the 4 posterior dental segments and the two anterior segments are the ones scored.

For example, teeth:

	16		21		27
47		41		35	

Before applying any stain to the deposits, the examiner first uses the naked eye to score the soft deposits, according to the following scale:

---

[1] The Oral Hygiene Index: A method for classifying oral hygiene status. J.A.D.A. 61, 171–179; 1957.

[2] The Simplified Oral Hygiene Index. J.A.D.A. 68, 7–13; 1964.

Oral debris (do not use your explorer!)

Grade 0: No soft deposits

Grade 1: Deposit or stain covers less than one-third of the tooth surface.

Grade 2: Deposits cover less than two-thirds of the surface.

Grade 3: Deposits cover more than two-thirds of the surface.

Example

Fig. VII-1

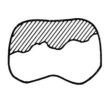 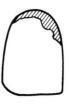 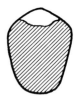

Tooth no. and surface	16 buccal	21 labial	35 lingual
Oral debris score	2	1	3

Dental calculus

Subsequently, the examiner uses the explorer to score the calculus deposits, again on the teeth with the most severe accumulations. The scores are as follows (see Fig. VII-2):

Grade 0: No calculus

Grade 1: Supragingival calculus covers less than one-third of the surface.

Grade 2: Supragingival calculus covers less than two-thirds of the surface, *or* single, isolated *sub*gingival calculus deposits.

Grade 3: Supragingival calculus covers more than two-thirds of the surface, *or subgin-* gival islands of calculus have fused to form a band around the neck of the tooth.

	<1/3	<2/3	islands	>2/3	band

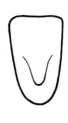 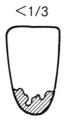 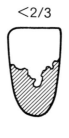 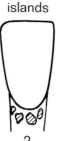 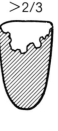 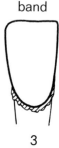

Fig. VII-2

Calculus score:	0	1	2	2	3	3

The OH-Plaque (oral debris) Index is scored per tooth, as the sum of the 12 scored surfaces divided by 6. The maximum score due to soft deposits is therefore 6 (3+3 for two surfaces).

The OH-Calculus Index is calculated in exactly the same manner. The greatest possible dental calculus score is thus also 6.

The total or combined OHI score is the sum of the plaque score plus the calculus score. The maximum OHI score is therefore 12! Moreover, since plaque and calculus are generally coexistent, the OHI score of 8 is seldom exceeded in practice.

Example

Relationship of the OHI score to the frequency of toothbrushing[1]
N = 188, subjects 26 to 32-years-old

Frequency of toothbrushing, per day	OHI
1 time	3.84
1	2.07
2	1.82
2	1.13

What should we think about when we see an OHI score of 3.84? Let's assume:

1. that the buccal and lingual plaque and calculus components were the same

$$\left(\frac{3.84}{2} = 1.92\right) \text{ and}$$

2. that *either* plaque *or* calculus was present on the tooth surfaces.

In this case, a score of 1.92 would mean that plaque or calculus covered approximately one-half of the facial and oral surfaces.

An OHI score of less than 2 has been regarded as "acceptable" oral hygiene, but OHI scores below 2.0 were found in only about 16% of the American population. 65% of the population had an OHI score of 2.1 to 5.9; 19% had scores of greater than 6.0!

OHI-Simplified, OHI-S

In this simplified OHI, the same criteria are used, but only six surfaces of six teeth are scored:

Buccal surfaces of teeth 16 and 26 (score second molars if first molars are missing)

Lingual surfaces of 36, 46 (37, 47 if first molars missing)

Labial surface of 41 (or 31)

Lingual surface of 31 (or 41)

[1] J. Periodont. 4, 14; 1969.

The maximum plaque index or the maximum calculus index would thus be 3, and the maximum OHI score would be 6. It is easy to understand, then, why, when reading OHI statistics, it is of the utmost importance to know whether OHI scores or OHI-S scores are being reported.

The Quigley-Hein Plaque Index

The QH Index is indicated for observation of oral hygiene measures, for example the cleaning efficacy of the toothbrush. The plaque is rendered visible through use of a staining solution (see page 138).

The determination is made from the stained facial and oral tooth surfaces (including transitional proximal surfaces).

Scoring

0 = absolutely no plaque

1 = single islands of plaque

2 = clear line of plaque along large extents of the gingival margin

3 = plaque on only the cervical third of the crown

4 = plaque extending into the middle third of the crown surface

5 = plaque into the occlusal third of the crown

Scores 2–5 are given even though the plaque is present on a mesial or distal portion only.

Examples

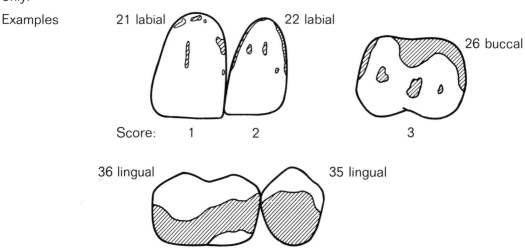

21 labial   22 labial   26 buccal

Score: 1   2   3

36 lingual   35 lingual

Score: 4   5   Fig. VII-3

During the scoring procedure, notice the differences in amount of plaque from surface to surface. One-third of the labial surface of a maxillary incisor is considerably wider than one-third of the lingual surface of a mandibular bicuspid!

Calculation: QH Index $= \dfrac{\text{sum of scores}}{\text{number of surfaces evaluated}}$

The Silness-Löe Plaque Index System[1]

The Quigley-Hein Index determined primarily the extent of deposits on the tooth surface. The thickness of the deposits was not considered. The QH Index also scored plaque which was far removed from the gingival margin and which therefore played no role in the etiology of gingivitis. On the other hand, the plaque index developed by Silness and Löe measures only the plaque immediately adjacent to the gingiva. The Silness-Löe index also attempts to consider the thickness of the plaque, because thickness is significantly related to gingivitis.

Procedure

Cervical plaque is scored in fully dentulous subjects, through use of the naked eye and an explorer, on three tooth surfaces. The surfaces to be considered are the mesial interdental area superior to the tip of the papilla, and the facial and oral survaces. *Do not stain the plaque!*

Depending upon the purpose of the investigation, scoring may be performed:

a) on all teeth

b) on half of the mouth

c) on selected teeth only.

Scoring criteria:

0 With good lighting, no plaque is visible adjacent to the marginal or papillary gingiva. Scraping with explorer also reveals no plaque.

1 A very thin microbial deposit near the marginal or papillary gingiva. When unstained, hardly visible to the naked eye. However, a scraping motion with the

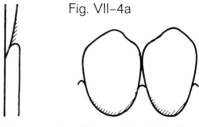

Fig. VII–4a

Score 1: hardly visible clinically

[1] Acta odont. scand. 22, 121; 1964.

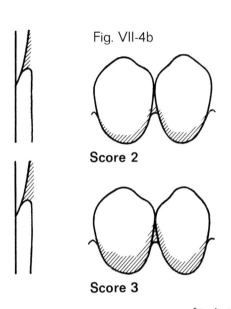

Fig. VII-4b

Score 2

Score 3

explorer on oral, facial and proximal surfaces removes plaque.

2 Soft deposits adjacent to the marginal gingiva and in the interdental area are easily visible. The interdental area is not completely filled with plaque.

3 A clearly visible, thick deposit is present adjacent to the gingival margin, and often extending far up the crown. The interdental space is completely filled with plaque.

Calculation: $\text{PI} = \dfrac{\text{sum of individual scores}}{\text{number of surfaces examined}}$

In our exercise, all surfaces of the crowns of teeth 16, 21, 24 and 44, 41, 36 will be evaluated. If any one of these teeth is missing, substitute its distal neighbor!

Plaque Planimetry

Under standardized conditions, color photographs are taken of stained plaque on one or several tooth surfaces. The negatives are projected onto white paper and the outline of the plaque is drawn. The "paper plaque" is then measured planimetrically, or it may be cut out and weighed. Both procedures are time-consuming and complicated, making the method applicable only for special investigations. See, for example, Kinoshita et al.[1] 1966 and Allet at al.[2] 1972.

Plaque Gravimetry

In this procedure, plaque is scraped with a plastic instrument from all tooth surfaces over a 5-minute interval. The plaque so obtained is collected and then weighed. When

[1] Kinoshita, S., Schait, A., Brebou, M., Mühlemann, H. R.: Effects of sucrose on early dental calculus and plaque. Helv. odont. Acta 10, 134–137; 1966.
[2] Allet, B., Regolati, B., Mühlemann, H. R.: Die Rolle der Griffabwinkelung auf die Reinigungskraft einer Zahnbürste. Schweiz. Mschr. Zahnheilk. 82, 452–460; 1972.

student-subjects stop all oral hygiene for 4 days, often 20–40 mg (wet weight) of plaque can be obtained per subject. The correlation between the results of a gravimetric plaque measurement and the Plaque Index of Silness-Löe is relatively close, as demonstrated by the graph[1] below.

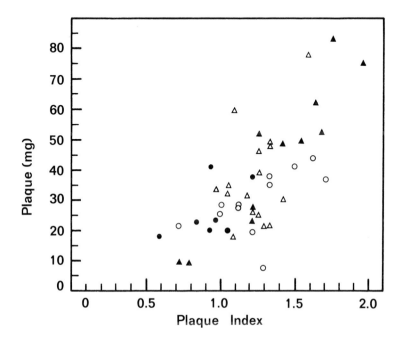

Fig. VII-5

[1] Scheinin, A., Mäkinen, K. K.: The effect of various sugars on the formation and chemical composition of dental plaque. Int. dent. J. 21, 302; 1971.

Additional literature

Bergenholtz, A.: Mechanical cleaning in oral hygiene. In: Oral Hygiene. Ed. A. Frandsen, Munksgaard, 1972, 27–62.

Ainamo, J.: Methods and means of evaluation of dental health programms. In: Oral Hygiene. Ed. A. Frandsen, Munksgaard, 1972, 139–154.

Elliott, J. R., Bowers, G. M.: I. Preventive periodontics utilizing an oral physiotherapy center. J. Periodontol. 43, 214; 1972.

Measurement of the Plaque

Subject: _____

Age: _____

Examiner: _____

Date: _____

1. Enter Pl (Silness-Löe) scores for teeth 16, 21, 24, 44, 41 and 36:

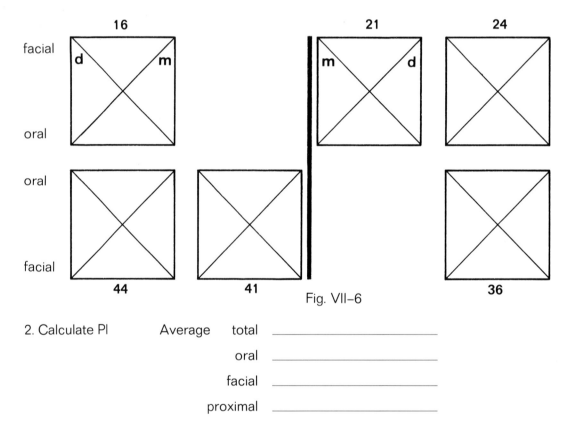

Fig. VII–6

2. Calculate Pl   Average   total   _____

                                    oral   _____

                                    facial   _____

                                    proximal _____

3. Stain the teeth with plaque disclosing solution. Try to
   distinguish between plaque and stained saliva coating (pellicle).
   Use your explorer with a scraping motion as well.

4. Enter QH Index for teeth 14, 11, 27, 47, 31, 34.

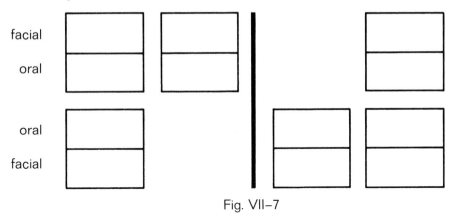

facial

oral

oral

facial

Fig. VII–7

5. Calculate the QH Index   Average   total _____
                                                     oral   _____
                                                     facial _____

Instructor's signature: _____

Measurement of the Plaque

Number of students: 23

Age: 23.6 ± 2.4 years   (range = 21 – 32)

1. Plaque Index of Silness-Löe

The determination was performed at about 10 o'clock in the morning, with no attempt having been made to alter the subjects' oral hygiene or eating habits.

Total PI = 0.58 ± 0.37 (0.04 – 1.30)

It would be interesting to make a comparision between these data and similar figures from Aarhus, Denmark, where the PI was developed. Are the Zurich students "cleaner"? Who would like to perform such a comparison?

In a separate study (winter semester 1972–73) on 19 subjects, the total PI was 0.62 ± 0.26, the facial PI was 0.30 ± 0.32, the lingual value was 0.58 ± 0.44, and the proximal score was 0.78 ± 0.32. How might these differences be explained?

2. Plaque Index of Quigley-Hein

QH = 1.58 ± 0.54   (range: 0.50 – 2.4)

The heaviest plaque accumulations were found on the most distal molars. The QHI was 2.1 ± 1.2 for the oral aspect of tooth 47, 1.8 ± 1.2 facially; for tooth 37 the lingual score was 1.6 ± 0.9, facial 2.3 ± 1.4. By comparison, for tooth 21, the labial score was 1.3 ± 1.0.

In another study on 18 subjects (winter semester 1972–73), the total QHI was 1.2 ± 0.64, lingually it was 1.43 ± 0.72 and facially 0.8 ± 0.64.

3. The degree of correlation between PI and QHI was +0.61; between QHI and CSI (Calculus Surface Index, see page 131), +0.46.

Dental Calculus Indices

1. Epidemiological studies (prevalence)

OH Index (OHI, Greene and Vermillion)

This index consists of a plaque (debris) component and a calculus component. We have already discussed it in terms of the OHI Plaque Index (see p. 121–122). It is not sensitive enough to measure small accumulations of calculus.

Ramfjord Calculus Index

This is one component of the Periodontal Disease Index (PDI) of Ramfjord (see Periodontal Disease – Epidemiology, Chapter X):

Grade 0: No calculus

Grade 1: Supragingival calculus approximately 1 mm in width at the cervical area

Grade 2: "Moderate" supragingival calculus and/or subgingival calculus

Grade 3: Abundant supra- and subgingival calculus

2. Incidence Studies

In studies of hygiene measures in patients, or during investigations of plaque or calculus inhibitory agents, the CSI or the VMI are usually employed.

CSI

Calculus Surface Index (1961)[1]

All four surfaces of the four mandibular incisors are evaluated. Only a yes–no determination for supra- and subgingival calculus is required. The CSI for each subject thus may be a maximum of 4x4 = 16. The length of time the calculus is dried prior to scoring influences the index results considerably. Drying time should always be the same: 15 seconds.

VM Index

Volpe and Manhold[2] presented this index in 1961 for evaluation of supragingival calculus. Several modifications have since been made. Using a graduated probe, the

---

[1] Ennever, J., Sturzenberger, O. P., and Radike, A. W.: The Calculus Surface Index method for scoring clinical calculus studies. J. Periodont. 32, 54; 1961.

[2] Volpe. A. R., and Manhold, J. H.: A method of evaluating the effectiveness of potential calculus inhibiting agents. N. Y. State Dent. J. 7, 289; 1962.

vertical extent of the calculus deposition on the lingual surfaces of the six mandibular anterior teeth is measured in millimeters in 3 locations. Calculus deposits less than 0.5 mm in extent are not recorded. Measurements are made as indicated in the figure below, i. e., at the median and the furthest lateral locations.

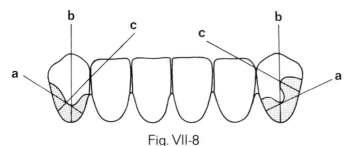

Sum of 3 measurements (a +b+c) = VMI of the tooth. The average of the 6 anterior teeth gives the VMI for the subject.

Fig. VII-8

MCL Index

The *Marginal Line Calculus Index*[1] was developed in 1967 for determination of calculus accumulation within a 1 to 2-week period. The extent of calculus is observed along the previously cleaned lingual gingival margin of the four mandibular incisor teeth. The marginal line is halved and the incidence is given in percent mesial and distal. The divisions are eighths. Anything less than 12.5% (⅛) is not recorded.

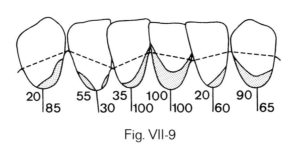

Fig. VII-9

Example: MCL index for the subject in Figure VII-9 =

$$\frac{20+85+55+30+35+100+100+100+20+60+90+65}{12} = 63\%$$

[1] Mühlemann, H. R. and Villa, P.: The Marginal Line Calculus Index. Helv. odont. Acta 11, 175; 1967.

Distribution of Calculus[1]

Upon which tooth surfaces does calculus most often accumulate?

Maximum ⟶ Minimum

Supragingival*	$\overline{1}$	$\overline{2}$	$\underline{6}$	$\underline{7}$	$\overline{3}$	$\overline{5}$	$\underline{5}$	$\overline{4}$	$\overline{6}$	$\overline{7}$	$\underline{1}$	$\underline{4}$	$\underline{2}$ $\underline{3}$
Subgingival	$\overline{1}$	$\underline{6}$	$\overline{6}$	$\underline{2}$	$\overline{7}$	$\underline{3}$	$\overline{4}$	$\overline{5}$	$\underline{7}$	$\underline{5}$	$\underline{2}$	$\underline{4}$	$\underline{3}$ $\underline{1}$
Proximal	$\overline{1}$	$\underline{2}$	$\underline{6}$	$\overline{3}$	$\overline{6}$	$\overline{4}$	$\overline{5}$	$\overline{7}$	$\underline{7}$	$\underline{5}$	$\underline{4}$	$\underline{2}$	$\underline{3}$ $\underline{1}$

The most interesting contrast is in the location of the supra- and subgingival calculus deposits upon the mandibular first molars as compared to those on the maxillary second molars.

Subgingival calculus is observed most often on the proximal surfaces; the lingual-marginal and buccal-marginal surfaces also are frequently sites of calculus deposition.[2]

* Numbers refer to teeth, e. g., 1 = incisor, 6 = first molar etc. Line *over* the number indicates a mandibular tooth; line *under* the number indicates a maxillary tooth.

[1] Ainamo, J.: Suom. Ham. Toim. 66, 301; 1970.

[2] Alexander, A. G.: A study of the distribution of supra and subgingival calculus, bacterial plaque and gingival inflammation in mouths of 400 individuals. J. Periodont. 42, 21; 1971.

Measurement of Dental Calculus

Subject: _____

Age: _____

Examiner: _____

Date: _____

1. Calculus Surface Index (CSI)

Dry the teeth for exactly 15 seconds. Perform your determinations using both eye and explorer.

42	41	31	32

$+$ = present

$-$ = absent

CSI = total number of surfaces with calculus

= _____

2. Volpe-Manhold Index (VMI)

Dry the lingual surfaces for 15 seconds. Perform determinations using a graduated probe. Make three measurements per lingual surface, and sum these values. Calculate the average of the sums for the 6 teeth. This gives the VM Index per subject.

43	42	41	−	31	32	33

mesial

median   VMI $\bar{x}_6$ = _____

distal

Instructor's signature: _____

Discussion of Exercise Results

1. Student groups of 23 and 18 subjects had average CSI scores of 7.13 ± 2.11 and 11.4 ± 3.5, respectively (data from 1971, 1972–73).

2. Average VMI scores of 1.25 ± 0.81 and 2.2 ± 0.9 were found in the same groups of 23 and 18 subjects, respectively.

It must be pointed out that these average results originated from as many examiners as there were subjects. Standard deviation values would demonstrate this.

The calculus indices of Greene and Vermillion and of Ramfjord were not performed in our exercise because they are not suitable for the determination of oral hygiene when it is as good as that usually found in dental students. Such indices are best employed to obtain a quick overview of the degree of oral cleanliness in a large group of subjects.

The VM Index is recommended for epidemiological prevalence studies, yet it is more often employed in incidence investigations. For example, a researcher may wish to test how much calculus builds up over a 2 to 4-month period in a test group vs a placebo group, when the test group has used some anti-calculus agent.

The CSI is a yes-or-no index, i. e., we determine whether or not calculus is present on the 16 surfaces of the four mandibular incisors. Very large variations exist among different examiners who have not been calibrated. The degree of variation will depend upon the care with which each investigator dries and assesses the surfaces under study. This is no doubt the origin of the large variations in the results of the two exercises shown above.

Additional example:

American investigations of calculus incidence showed the CSI to increase from zero to approximately 5.6 – 7.7 over an 8-week period. In Zurich, a score of 7.5 had already been attained in only one week. It is improbable that Zurich citizens "calcify" so much more quickly! Probably, more time was given to examination, and even very tiny calcified deposits were scored as "yes" surfaces during the latter study.

The MLC Index, which we did not perform in our exercises, makes it possible to estimate the rate of calculus deposition after only one week of observation. Experience has proven that a plateau is reached in supragingival calculus deposition on the lingual surfaces of lower incisor teeth after two weeks. For this reason, it is senseless to try to use the MLCI over long periods of time to test the efficacy of anti-calculus agents.

Foil technique[1]

This method of determining the rate of calculus formation was developed in Zurich. Roughened Mylar plastic foils of standardized size are fastened to the cleaned lingual surfaces of mandibular incisors using nylon thread. The foils are allowed to remain in situ for 7 to 14 days. Calculus which accumulates during this period is weighed with the removed foil and analyzed for its calcium, phosphorus and fluoride content. In addition, foils may be prepared for histological examination, thus permitting morphological observations (both light and electron microscopy) as well as chemical and physical (e. g., x-ray diffraction) findings. The various types of findings can then be compared and correlated. For insight into recent investigations, read about the anti-calculus effectiveness of diphosphonates[2].

Reports about percentage reductions of calculus formation by whatever agents should be viewed with reserve, as evidenced by the following example[3]:

Calculus inhibition was studied in 18 student-subjects who used a mouthwash for 11 weeks. Three different indices were employed, in addition to the foil method. The resulting "percentage reduction" data are summarized in the Table below.

Index	Length of study	Placebo group	Test group	Percentage reduction
VM	1	0.3	0.1	74
	5	1.1	1.0	9
	11	1.2	1.4	−18 (increase!)
CS	1	7.5	6.8	10
	5	9.6	7.9	18
	11	10.2	9.6	6
MLC	1	50.0	37.7	25
	5	–	61.4	–
	11	74.3	68.2	8
Foils μg	1	1064	761	28

[1] Mühlemann, H. R., Schroeder, H. E. in: Advances in Oral Biology. Dynamics of Supragingival Calculus Formation. P. H. Staple, 1964.

[2] Mühlemann, H. R. et al.: Effect of diphosphonate on human supragingival calculus. Helv. odont. Acta 14, 31; 1970.

[3] Villa, P. R. et al.: A comparison of various calculus incidence indices. Helv. odont. Acta 11, 180; 1967.

It becomes clear how much the reduction figures depend upon the type of index used and the length of the study. It is advisable to perform a preliminary one-week test with the foil method, then to follow up with a long-term study (3 to 4 months) using the VM Index. A very important factor influencing the rate of calculus accumulation is the smoothness of the surface upon which the calculus accumulation is taking place. Plaque accumulates much more rapidly upon rough surfaces than upon smooth ones, and mineralization leads quickly to formation of calculus.

Mineralization Anesthesia:

   Gram-positive bugs sat content,
   Secure in an enamel dent.
    But by membrane penetration
    They experienced mineralization:
   To sleep like van Winkel they went!

Plaque Disclosing Agents (Plaque detectors)

Synonyms: Disclosing solutions, plaque staining solutions, disclosing wafers.

As early as 1943, Raybin[1] recognized that making dental plaque visible could be of significance both in motivating patients toward better oral hygiene, and in helping them to reach a higher standard of home care. It was not until 1959, however, that Arnim[2] really introduced the world to plaque disclosing solutions.

A plaque detector is a coloring agent which is either painted onto the teeth by the dentist or is used at home by the patient. Where home use is concerned, plaque detectors are incorporated in a mouthwash or in a tablet which is chewed up and swished around the oral cavity. During the last 10 years, the three agents most often used for plaque disclosing in the dental office have been basic fuchsin, mercurochrome® and neutral red. Earlier iodine-potassium iodide, gentian violet and crystal violet were in vogue. It was Hueper[3], in 1959, who proposed the disclosing tablet containing F.D.C. Red # 3 (erythrosin) for home use.

Plaque detectors should selectively stain bacteria but NOT the oral fluid or the mucosa. They must not be poisonous and must not be sensitizing agents. They must not adhere to filling materials which are free of plaque, and must not permanently stain clothing or skin. Unfortunately, the ideal disclosing agent has yet to be found.

Staining Agents

1. Basic fuchsin (Synonyms include basic violet, rosanaline, magenta)

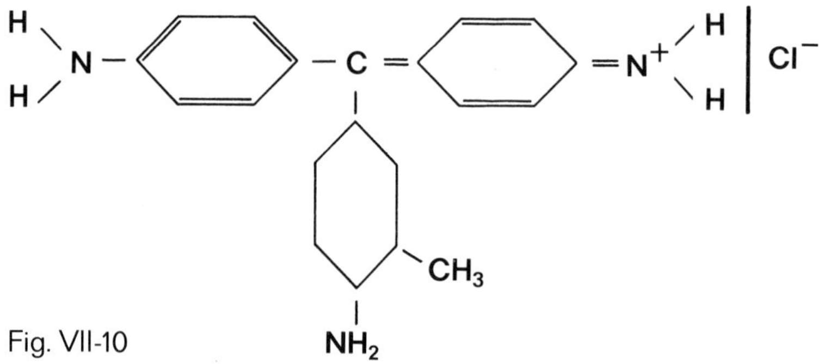

Fig. VII-10

Although this substance is only slightly soluble in water, it is readily soluble in ethyl alcohol. Used as a disclosing solution it is neither toxic nor carcinogenic*. The oral LD_{50}

---

[1] All numbered literature references will be found on page 142.

* R. A. M. Case, Chester Beatty Institute, London. Personal communication.

in rabbits is 150 mg/kg. Nonetheless, there is still some commotion about the use of basic fuchsin as a disclosing agent*.

The dentist applies basic fuchsin at a concentration of 2%. The patient may also use it as a 1% rinsing solution.

Rx   Basic fuchsin   1.5
        Spiritus   25.0

Disp. dropper bottle

Sig. As a mouthrinse: Approx. 15 drops per 1/4 glass of water

2. Mercurochrome or merbromine as a 5% solution. This is a mercury-containing disinfectant which is applied by the dentist.

3. Erythrosin (F.D.C. Red # 3)

For topical application:
Apply a 5% solution by means of a cotton-tipped applicator to the teeth and rinse lightly with a water stream.

For rinsing:
Apply 6 drops of a 5% solution to the tongue and "rinse."

As a disclosing tablet: 15 mg/tablet

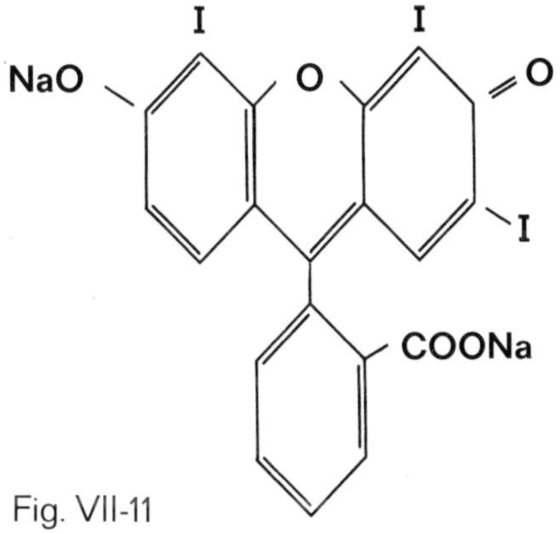

Fig. VII-11

Erythrosin has been accepted as an additive in food, medicines, cosmetics and disclosing tablets by the United States Food and Drug Administration (F.D.A.), known to be one of the most strict regulatory agencies. Disclosing tablets, containing 15 mg of erythrosin plus binders and aromatics, have been used very widely in the United States since the early 1960's. It is expressly stated that these tablets may be swallowed after they have been chewed up[4,5]. The intraperitoneal LD_{50} is 300 mg/kg for rats. If a 5 to 6-year-old child swallows an erythrosin tablet, the dose[6] per kilogram body weight is 0.75 mg/kg. Erythrosin does, however, contain iodine! Therefore, the possibility of iodine allergy must be kept in mind. Even though erythrosin tablets have been more and more widely used over the past 10 years, in organized school programs as well as in pedodontic dental practice, there have been – as far as this author knows – no published reports of deleterious side effects, except for one allergic reaction. It is recommended that the oral fluid be expectorated after an erythrosin disclosing wafer is used. But this recommendation is more for psychological reasons than for toxicological ones.

* H. L. Küng, Ciba-Geigy AG. Personal communication.

4. Proflavin

BOFORS-Nobel-Pharma in Sweden also makes disclosing tablets. Theirs contain 2.5 mg of the yellow coloring agent Proflavin. The BOFORS tablets has not found wide acceptance among continental Europeans.

5. Malachite Green
   (synonyms: Victoria green, fast green, F.D.C. green # 3)

Malachite green is chemically very closely related to basic fuchsin. Details concerning biological and toxic effects have been reviewed by Werth (see ref. 7). Topical application of a 1.0–2.5% solution provides good staining of plaque and a good contrast with the pink gingiva as well.

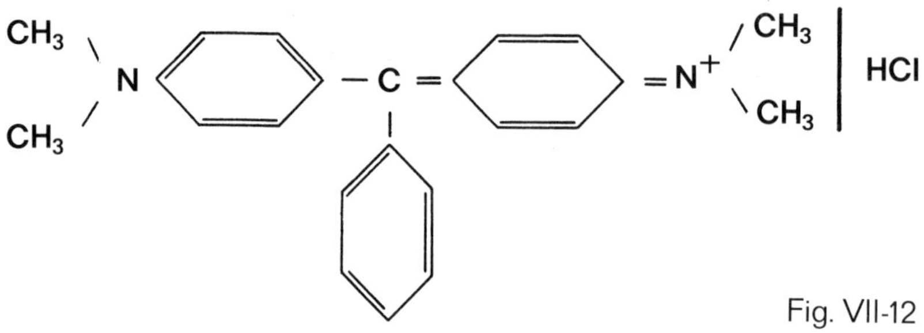

Fig. VII-12

Malachite green is not supposed to influence the growth of plaque microorganisms, but the evidence is not yet conclusive. This agent will not become a widely used disclosing substance because of its theoretical toxicity: the oral LD_{50} in rabbits is 75 mg/kg.

The same is true of the other triphenylmethane derivatives, gentian violet (methyl violet) and crystal violet[8].

In the future, food coloring agents will become the disclosing agents of choice. Several of these, such as erythrosin, have been shown to be well suited for this purpose.

6. Tartrazine
   (= hydrazine yellow, see Fig. VII-13, p. 141) and Patent Blue V (see ref. 8)

Both substances are permitted as food coloring in Switzerland (pistachio green). For plaque disclosure, they are mixed in the ratio of 85 : 15, tartrazine-to-patent blue, the mixture having been prepared as a 4% water solution.

Tartrazin

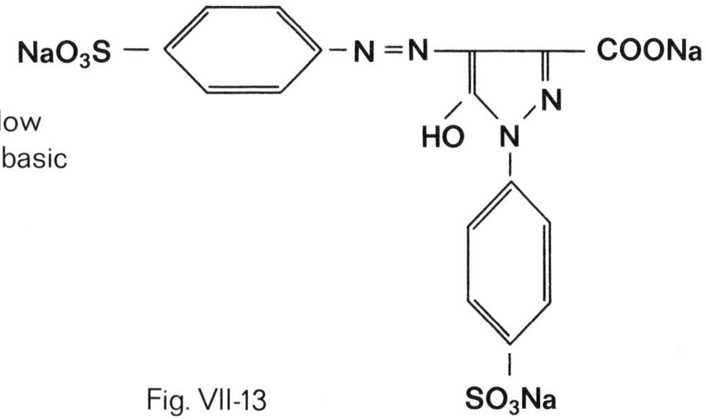

Coloring agent, orange-yellow
at pH 7.1. Becomes red in basic
solution.

Fig. VII-13

Patent Blue is a tri-aryl methane

Recently, these two coloring agents became commercially available in Switzerland as a solution called "Chromoplak." This product stains dental plaque nicely green[9], and does not stain the layer of denatured saliva which is so often adherent to teeth, gingiva and tongue. Chromoplak lacks the staining effectiveness of basic fuchsin, however. On the other hand, it disappears more quickly from the oral cavity, which is considered an advantage.

Recently in the United States, a disclosing solution (DIS-PLAQUE) has come onto the market which contains a combination of F.D.C.-approved colors. Older, thicker plaque is supposed to stain blue, while young, thin plaque (exogenous enamel cuticle!) is stained a reddish color. Staining power is good.

Fluorescent plaque detectors

Most coloring agents also stain the bacteria on the tongue and other areas of the oral cavity a red color which lasts for hours. It is therefore preferable to use these plaque detectors just before going to bed.

The fluorescent substances attempt to do away with the cosmetic disadvantages of disclosing solutions. A new plaque control system employs the "plaque-o-philic" agent sodium fluorescein, which glows yellow when illuminated with a special blue light source (PLAK-LITE), but which is invisible in normal daylight.

It has been shown[10] that the fluorescing solution* selectively stains the plaque. Exogenous enamel cuticle, gingiva, mucosal surfaces and clean teeth do not fluoresce.

---

* Packaging: $\frac{1}{2}$ fluid ounce dropper bottle containing 0.75% solution of D. & C. Yellow No. 8 (Na-Fluorescein)

The correlation of the fluorescent findings with the Silness-Löe Plaque Index is practically linear if the PI is > 0.5. In patients with only very little plaque, no correlation exists. (Staining with erythrosin reveals somewhat larger stained areas than does fluorescein staining.) Plaque growth is not influenced by sodium fluorescein. The solution is well accepted by patients. The taste is not unpleasant and the fluorescence disappears completely after two hours.

One disadvantage of the PLAK-LITE is its high cost. Also, the test can be performed only in the dark.

Literature

[1] Raybin, M.: Disclosing solutions, their importance and uses. D. Outlook 30, 149; 1943.

[2] Arnim, S. S.: Microcosms of the human mouth. J. Tenn. D. A. 39, 3; 1959.

[3] Hueper, W. C., Chief, Environmental Cancer Section, National Cancer Institute, N. I. H., Bethesda, Md.; see Arnim, S. S.: the use of disclosing agents for measuring tooth cleanliness. J. Periodont. 34, 227; 1963.

[4] Arnim, S. S.: The use of disclosing agents for measuring tooth cleanliness. J. Periodont. 34, 227; 1963

[5] Arnim, S. S. et al.: What you need to know and do to prevent dental caries and periodontal disease. North Carolina Dent. Soc. 46, 340; 1963.

[6] Handbook of Toxicology. Vol. I, Ed. W. S. Spector. W. B. Saunders, London 1956.

[7] Fundak, C. P., Ash, M. M.: Pilot investigation of correlations between supragingival plaque, subgingival plaque and gingival crevice depth. J. Periodont. 40, 20; 1969.

[8] Bouquet, P.: Colorants et détection de la plaque dentaire. Rev. franç. odonto-stomatol. 18, 1239; 1971.

[9] Lang, N. P., Østergaard, E., and Löe, H.: A fluorescent plaque disclosing agent. J. Periodont. Res. 7, 59–67; 1962.

[10] Hansen, F., Gjermo, P.: The plaque-removing effect of four toothbrushing methods. Scand. J. dent. Res. 79, 502; 1071.

[11] Cohen, D. W. et al.: A comparison of bacterial plaque disclosants in periodontal disease. J. Periodont. 43, 333; 1972.

Gingivitis

Instruction Sheets

VIII-1: Epidemiology of gingival inflammation

VIII-2: Crevicular fluid

Exercise and Data Sheets

VIII-1: The Sulcus Bleeding Index

VIII-2: Measurement of crevicular fluid

Results Sheets

VIII-1: SB Index

VIII-2: Crevicular fluid

Material

Student: cotton pliers, mouth mirror, explorer, periodontal probe

Instructor: filter paper strips, microscope slides, ninhydrin, millimeter rules, Scotch tape, sodium fluorescein for injection 20%. Injection syringe. UV lamp.

Program

1. Discussion of results from Exercise VII, "Oral Hygiene"

2. Introduction to today's topic

3. Exercises

Epidemiology of Gingival Inflammation

Morbidity is too gross a criterion for differentiating the prevalence of gingivitis in one population from that in another. A study in Zurich[1] in 1957, for example, revealed that 85% of 14-year-olds already had inflamed gingiva. The same, you will recall, was found to be the case when dental caries was expressed by morbidity.

Gingivitis prevalence

The term gingivitis prevalence means the number of inflamed gingival units in the oral cavity at any one time. It does not necessarily signify the "lifetime gingivitis experience," as was the case with caries, which increases with time because of its irreversibility. Gingivitis can regress, at least in part, so gingivitis indices are to a certain extent reversible. "Reversals" which occur in the DMF index (for example a tooth surface may be scored D_2 at the initial examination and D_0 six months later) are almost always the result of method error and do not represent true reversibility.

Massler et al.[2], in 1950, introduced the gingival units:

M = Marginal gingiva

P = Papillary gingiva

A = Attached gingiva.

In the Massler PMA Index, the inflamed, i. e., the clearly reddened, swollen, spontaneously bleeding or ulcerated facial P, M and A's per dentition, dental arch, or quadrant, are counted.

Thus: 1 – 3 inflamed gingival units per dentition is taken to be "mild gingivitis" and

7 – 12 inflamed gingival units per dentition is termed "severe gingivitis."

Inflamed "M" is considered more serious than inflamed "P."

[1] Mazor, Z. S.: Gingivitis bei Zürcher Schulkindern. Med. Diss., Zürich 1958.
[2] Massler, M., Schour, J., Copra, B.: Occurrences of gingivitis in children. J. Periodont. 21, 146; 1950.

For similar reasons, the Rosenzweig[1] modification of the PMA Index gives numerical values of 1,2 and 3 to the P, M and A gingival units, respectively.

PMA scores obtained with the Massler Index are only meaningful if the reader knows how many gingival units have been examined and if the PMA score is given with both the single constituent values and the total (e. g., PMA score = 12: 7P, 4M, 1A).

Gingivitis incidence

The Massler PMA Index in its original form served as the basis for numerous epidemiological prevalence studies in many different countries. But the Massler Index is not sensitive enough to detect differences among individuals or groups with regard to gingivitis incidence, increment (increase in gingivitis) or decrement (decrease in gingivitis). Accordingly, if one wishes to measure the effectiveness of a particular therapeutic or preventive measure, or to investigate the influence of marginal irritation, the Massler PMA Index is not the index to use. The original PMA index was modified and refined by Mühlemann and Mazor[2] in 1956. In 1963, Löe and Silness[3] and in 1967 Löe[4] alone proposed the Gingival Index System for much the same reasons.

The SB Index

On the European continent, the Massler PMA Index is used almost exclusively in its Mühlemann modification. In principle, this modification expresses not only the number of inflamed gingival P and M units in a dentition, but also the severity of the inflammation of these units. In order to avoid confusion, the Mühlemann modification of the original Massler PMA Index has recently been termed the Sulcus Bleeding Index[5] because bleeding from the sulcus is the first clinically detectable sign of gingival inflammation. The bleeding which follows gentle probing of the gingival sulcus represents the initial and leading symptom of initial gingivitis. Other signs, such as the reddening, swelling or discoloration of the gingival margin or papilla, occur only later and are more difficult to define. The SB Index is identical to the previously used PMA Index as modified by Mühlemann.

[1] Rosenzweig, K. H.: Gingivitis in children of Israel. J. Periodont. 31, 404; 1960.

[2] Mühlemann, H. R. and Mazor, Z. S.: Gingivitis in Zurich school children. Helv. odont. Acta 2, 3; 1958.

[3] Löe, H., Silness, J.: Periodontal disease in pregnancy. Acta odont. Scand. 21, 533; 1963.

[4] Löe, H.: Gingival index, the plaque index and the retention index systems. J. Periodont. 38, 610; 1967.

[5] Mühlemann, H. R., Son, S.: Gingival sulcus bleeding–a leading symptom in initial gingivitis. Helv. odont. Acta 15, 107; 1971.

Scoring inflammation with the SB Index

Grade 0

Healthy appearing P and M units. *No* bleeding upon careful, blunt probing of the gingival sulcus.

Grade 1

Healthy appearing P and M units, without discoloration or swelling. But, upon careful, blunt probing of the gingival sulcus or pocket, tiny bleeding points appear after 1 – 15 seconds.

Grade 2

Bleeding subsequent to probing of the sulcus, *and* inflammatory color alterations of P and M units. No swelling or macroscopic edema.

Grade 3

Bleeding subsequent to probing, *and* color alterations, *and* slight edematous swelling of P and M units.

Grade 4

a) Bleeding upon sulcus probing *and* color alterations *and* obvious swelling, or

b) Bleeding upon sulcus probing *and* obvious swelling (no color changes).

Grade 5

Bleeding upon sulcus probing, *and* spontaneous bleeding *and* color alterations; severe swelling with or without ulceration.

In the SB Index, we do not score the A gingival unit (attached gingiva) because it is involved only very seldom in the European population.

The Gingival Index System (GI)

The GI is applicable for prevalence and incidence studies, just as is the SBI. It is very popular in Scandinavia, in spite of the fact that it is less sensitive than the SB Index. The GI ignores Grade 1 of the SBI. The GI Grade 1 corresponds approximately to the SBI Grade 2. Decreased sensitivity of the GI in comparison to the SBI has been reported[1]. The results may be summarized as follows:

---

[1] Alexander, A. G.: An assessment of the inter- and intraexaminer agreement in scoring gingivitis clinically. J. Periodont. Res. 6, 146; 1971.

13 students ceased all oral hygiene measures for 17 days. A total of 832 P and M gingival units were evaluated using the SBI and the GI.

Frequency of inflammation Grades 0–3 on P and M gingival units

Index used	Grade	Beginning of study	End of study	Comment
SBI	0	738	264	marked decrease
	1	88	470	marked increase
	2	6	89	
	3	0	9	
GI	0	826	734	slight decrease!
	1	6	89	slight increase!
	2	0	9	

Helv. odont. Acta 15, 107; 1971.

Any evaluation of gingivitis is dependent to a greater or lesser degree upon the examiner's subjective interpretations. Nonetheless, if investigators are calibrated before a study is undertaken, the variation among them is not significant. The bleeding symptom is a consistent parameter.

The Sulcus Bleeding Index (SBI)

Depending upon the goal of the investigation, it is often sufficient to determine the SB index on the facial M and P gingival units only. The oral surface values may also be useful in some instances. For the purposes of this exercise, we will determine the SBI on 6 areas per tooth. The areas through which the probe should move are indicated by thickened lines in Figure VIII-1 (below).

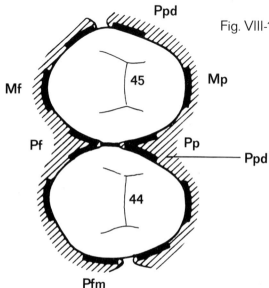

Fig. VIII-1: Pf = facial papilla, Pp = palatal papilla

Areas to be probed (dark lines):
Mf – facial marginal gingiva
Mp – palatal marginal gingiva
Pfm – mesiofacial papilla
Pdp – distopalatal papilla

Sulcus probing is performed with a fine yet blunt periodontal probe, using a force of about 20–30 P[1]. The probe is carefully inserted into the sulcus, until slight resistance is encountered. The probe tip is then moved laterally back and forth a distance of 3 to 4 mm as indicated in Figure VIII-1 (thick, dark lines).

Class partners should first pracitce "gentle" probing, then definitively determine the Sulcus Bleeding Index, and enter results in the chart on page 149 (Fig. VIII-2). Choose the maxillary quadrant with the least number of fillings. Determine SBI on incisors, cuspid, bicuspids and first molar.

---

[1] Gabathuler, H., Hassell, T.: A pressure-sensitive periodontal probe. Helv. odont. Acta 15, 114; 1971.

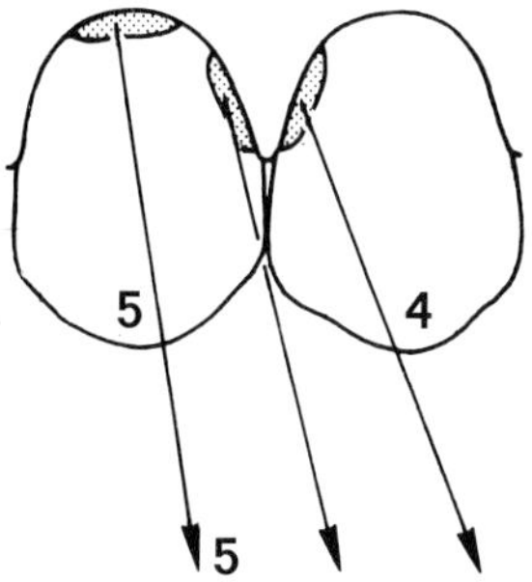

Subject: ____________________

Examiner: ____________________

Date: ____________________

	5			4			3			2			1		
	P	M	P	P											
facial															
palatal															
	d	m											Pd	M	Pm

Tooth 6

	dP	M	mP	dP	M	mP
facial						
palatal	dP		M		mP	

(mesial and distal buccal roots)

Fig. VIII-2

1. Check one: upper right [ ] left [ ]. Cross out missing teeth! Perform probing, then enter gingivitis score, including zeros (wait 15 seconds for bleeding points).

2. Calculate average SB indices (sum of single values divided by the number of examined units):

SBI total	N = ________	$\bar{x}$ = ________
SBI palatal	N = ________	$\bar{x}$ = ________
SBI facial	N = ________	$\bar{x}$ = ________
SBI papillary	N = ________	$\bar{x}$ = ________
SBI marginal	N = ________	$\bar{x}$ = ________

3. What percent of examined units are inflamed? ________

Instructor's signature: ____________________

SB Index

The SB index was used to evaluate 39 gingival units around six teeth (central incisor up to and including first molar) in 28 subjects. Two subjects were completely free of inflammation in the areas examined. The gingivitis morbidity of the group was thus 93%.

The average gingivitis prevalence was:

SBI			Range
total	$\bar{x}$ =	0.26 ± 0.27	0.0– 1.24
palatal	$\bar{x}$ =	0.24 ± 0.23	0.0– 0.13
facial	$\bar{x}$ =	0.27 ± 0.35	0.0– 1.60
papillary	$\bar{x}$ =	0.31 ± 0.32	0.0– 1.40
marginal	$\bar{x}$ =	0.14 ± 0.18	0.0– 0.80
			0.0–91.00

In comparison:

GI papillary	0.06 ± 0.12
GI marginal	0.04 ± 0.15

Of the 39 units at risk, 22.3 $\pm$ 20.0% were affected according to the SB index (9–10 units).

The percent of Grades 1- and 2-units was 20.5%.

The percent of Grade 2-units was 4.8%.

These last two figures make it clear that the morbidity is quite dependent upon the definition of gingivitis. This was shown in the investigations by Mühlemann and Mazor[1].

Gingivitis morbidity* in Zurich schoolchildren

Age	SBI Grade 1 scored	SBI Grade 1 not scored. (Initial sign of inflamation was thus gingival reddening)
7	75	15
8	88	36
9	89	37
15	88	40

* expressed as a percentage.

[1] Mühlemann, H. R. and Mazor, S.: Helv. Odont. Acta 2, 3; 1958.

In this study, 22 units in the anterior region were examined. Approximately ⅓ of the units exhibited inflammatory alterations. There were differences with regard to sex and age.

Average number of diseased P and M units, as scored with the SB index (number of teeth at risk = 22)

Age in years	Boys	Girls
9	6.7	7.3
10	6.7	7.3
11	7.0	9.4
12	7.6	8.7
13	9.0	8.2
14	6.5	6.3

SB Index:

> The gingiva screamed, mad as hell:
> "Plaque deposits do not do me well.
> I did all I could
> But with probing comes blood,
> And my tender papillae do swell"!

Crevicular Fluid

Synonyms: sulcus fluid, gingival fluid, sulcus exudate, pocket exudate.

Definition

The crevicular fluid (CF) is an inflammatory, cell-containing exudate. No such fluid exits from the clinically healthy gingiva. As the severity of inflammation increases, so does the amount of crevicular exudate. For this reason, measurement of the rate of flow of this crevicular fluid is one way of determining the degree of inflammation.

The physiological function of crevicular fluid is to rinse away catabolites. It contains protective elements, but it may also serve as a nutritive substrate for some bacteria. Sodium fluorescein injected i–v, or tetracycline taken orally will be transported via the circulatory system to the gingival sulcus area, and these substances can be demonstrated in the crevicular fluid.

Determination of CF

CF is measured by the use of standardized filter paper strips, 8.3 x 1.25 mm in size. The lower end of each strip is either placed at the entrance to the gingival sulcus (this placement is called the extracrevicular method) or is inserted into the sulcus until light resistance is encountered (the intracrevicular method). The strips are allowed to remain in situ for three minutes.

For quantitative evaluation, the strips are soaked with a ninhydrin solution. In the presence of crevicular fluid, a chemical reaction turns the amino acids a blue color, so that the portion of the filter paper strip which has soaked up crevicular fluid can be planimetrically or longitudinally measured.

The diagrams on the following page illustrate both methods, as well as the measurement of the stained strips.

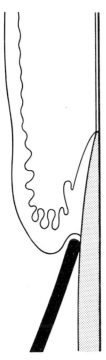

Extracrevicular method (strip is positioned in the histological sulcus)

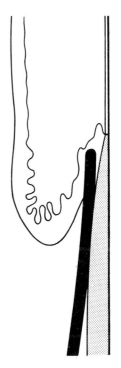

Intracrevicular method (strip positioned in the clinical sulcus)

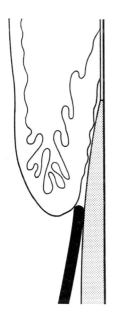

Fig. VIII-3

Extracrevicular method in the case of a periodontal pocket

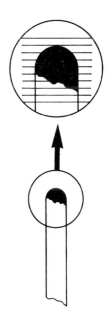

Determination of crevicular fluid using a hand lens (the horizontal lines are graduated)

153

Measurement of Crevicular Fluid

Subject: _____

Examiner: _____

Date: _____

1. Measurement by means of the intracrevicular method

Method: Place cotton rolls and dry the area gently with an air stream. Insert the strip until it bends ever so slightly because it has met slight resistance.

With the aid of a stop watch, leave the strip in place for 3 minutes. Remove the strip, using a sharp pointed explorer. Pierce the strip with the explorer point exactly at the gingival margin, and you will have thus marked the depth to which the strip was inserted. Attach the various strips to a microscope slide using Scotch tape. Write the subject's name and the tooth number on the slide. You are now ready to stain with ninhydrin.

Position of the strip   Strip removal

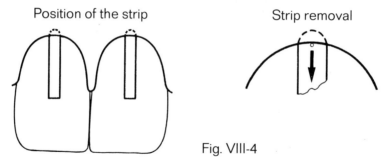

Fig. VIII-4

2. Comparison of clinical inflammation and crevicular fluid

Choose two proximal areas which are clinically free of inflammation and two which are inflamed (look in the neighborhood of rough filling margins or where plaque is evident). Now proceed to measure crevicular fluid flow rate at these four sites. After the strips have been in place for three minutes, mount them on a microscope slide for staining. Then determine SBI scores around these teeth. Fill in the chart below.

Proximal areas between teeth	SBI of the P unit	Sulcus depth mesial distal	Amount of crevicular fluid collected from P unit mesial distal
_____	_____	_____ _____	_____ _____
_____	_____	_____ _____	_____ _____
_____	_____	_____ _____	_____ _____
_____	_____	_____ _____	_____ _____

3. Proof of the origin of crevicular fluid

Several subjects will have 2 ml of a 20% sodium fluorescein solution injected i-v into a vein of the cubital fossa immediately before the crevicular fluid measurements are to be made. In the case of these subjects, insert the strips into sulci which have inflamed P or M units. Be very careful to prevent contamination of the strips with oral fluid. The strips should be left in situ for 3 minutes, then removed and examined under a UV-light in a darkened room.

Instructor's signature: _____

Crevicular Fluid

In an earlier investigation with 13 students, SBI and crevicular fluid flow rate were determined at the end of a phase of intensive oral hygiene and subsequently during 17 days without oral hygiene measures[1].

	Day 0	3	6	10	13	17
Mean SBI	0.12	0.10	0.43	0.60	0.76	0.81
Mean crevicular fluid flow rate, in mm	0.49	0.97	1.19	1.17	1.26	1.64

Each time a strip is inserted into a completely healthy sulcus, as seen clinically, the epithelium is torn and tissue fluid from this microwound is absorbed by the strip. For this reason, if the intracrevicular method is employed, a strip may be irregularly stained even when it has been within an inflammation-free sulcus. The staining of the strip which appears under these circumstances can be disregarded because it is created by tissue fluid, rather than by inflammatory exudate.

The demonstration with sodium fluorescein could not be performed because of the low SBI scores. There were no severely reddened and swollen PM units present. In a subsequent exercise, we will attempt to demonstrate the intracrevicular release of i–v injected sodium fluorescein around inflamed gingiva in a patient with active periodontal disease.

Sulcus Fluid:

> The dental papilla was mad:
> "I'm swollen and wet and that's sad!
>   'Cause one thing I know
>   Is that sulcular flow
> Hygienically speaking, is bad"!

---

[1] Mühlemann, H. R., Son, S.: Gingival Sulcus Bleeding–a leading symptom in initial gingivitis. Helv. odont. Acta 15, 107; 1971.

Iatrogenic Marginal Irritation

Instruction Sheet

IX-1: Iatrogenic marginal irritants

Exercise Sheet

IX-1: Iatrogenic marginal irritants

Result Sheet

IX-1: Discussion of exercise results

Material

Student: mirror, short and long explorers, periodontal probe, separator, dental floss.
            Student's own radiographic survey
Instructor: x-ray viewbox

Program

1. Discussion of results from Exercise VIII

2. Introduction to today's topic

3. Exercises

Iatrogenic Marginal Irritants

"Iatrogenic marginal irritation" is nothing more than a nice name for a sad chapter in therapeutic medicine. Iatros = doctor.

Treatment, in the sense of filling a carious defect with a restoration which duplicates exactly the previously existing tooth morphology is simply not possible, despite all the technological progress to date.

Irritations may result from mistakes made during restorative procedures and may be of occlusal or of marginal nature.

Occlusal irritations or trigger zones are created by disharmonies in centric and lateral occlusion. Filling material may interfere during the closing and/or the lateral movements of the jaw. These premature contacts or lateral interferences can have pathological consequences for the entire oral system.

Marginal irritations (irritations of the gingival margin) are more severe and occur more often.

Below are some examples of marginal irritants:

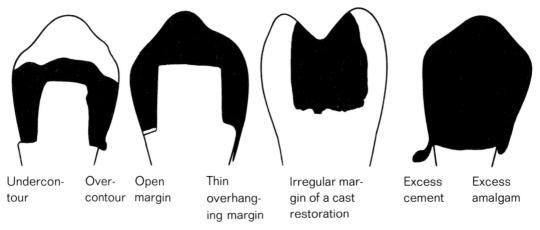

| Undercon-
tour | Over-
contour | Open
margin | Thin
overhang-
ing margin | Irregular mar-
gin of a cast
restoration | Excess
cement | Excess
amalgam |

Fig. IX-1

Achieving perfect cervical and proximal fillings and cervical crown margins is a high art. Every situation which leads to plaque retention causes gingival inflammation and/or secondary caries. Such situations include: undercontour, overcontour and rough surfaces of filling materials, as well as filling material debris in the interdental space, open and irregular crown margins, food impaction due to improper occlusal morphology, and incorrect placement of interdental contact areas.

A frightening look at reality

1. Oral uncleanliness, high sugar intake, fluoride deficiences and ignorance lead rapidly to

2. carious occlusal lesions. These are then

3. treated and filled, with inclusion of the still-sound proximal surfaces, in the name of "extension for prevention(!)."

4. Unavoidable imperfections in the proximal cervical region of the restorations quickly cause a papillitis, and by way of plaque retention often lead to secondary caries as well. This requires

5. a new treatment session for caries.

6. In an attempt at caries prevention(!), the treatment is performed using a gold crown, which is supposed to prevent cervical caries because the crown margin is located far beneath the free gingival margin. This concept, introduced by G.V.Black as "extension for prevention of caries," is also known in Norway today, but by a different phrase: "extension for the promotion of periodontal disease"[1]. In reality, the consequences of this type of gold crown-caries prevention are often as follows:
   - High cost, which may, however, be gladly accepted by patients because gleaming gold crowns are often social status symbols.
   - Intensive marginal irritation, due to open crown margins, or—even more frequently–due to cement debris which remain in the interdental area after the crown is seated. This initiates the development of periodontal pockets.

With time, additional consequences may result from treatment for dental caries. These include:

7. Pulp necrosis due to mechanical and chemical pulp damage stemming from preparation of the tooth for the crown. This may lead to

8. pulpal and/or periapical abscesses. Thereafter, conservative and surgical attempts at root canal therapy sometimes lead to

9. tooth extraction. Tooth loss nececcitates

10. grinding upon the adjacent teeth in order to prepare them to receive the abutment crowns of a bridge replacement for the extracted tooth. And here new complications arise; begin again at number 7, above.

[1] Wearhaug, J.: Needs and potentials for clinical research in periodontology. J. Periodont. 40, 155; 1969.

Modern therapeutic cariology recommends more and more vehemently that all filling and crown margins be placed supragingivally[1]. Sometimes this requires that gingival surgery be performed (usually simple papillectomies).

The diagnosis of iatrogenic, marginal irritation in not easy. Irritants, be they subgingival or supragingival, can be reliably diagnosed only on a clinical basis, through use of the dental explorer and direct vision. A radiographically evident irritation is always present clinically, but the reverse need not be true! Many plastic filling materials are not visible at all in the radiograph.

[1] Renggli, H. H.: Auswirkungen subgingivaler approximaler Füllungsränder auf den Entzündungsgrad der benachbarten Gingiva. Schweiz. Mschr. Zahnheilk. 83, 10; 1974.

Iatrogenic Marginal Irritations

Subject: _____

Examiner: _____

Date: _____

1. Frequency of radiographically-evident imperfections (irritants)

On your own radiographic survey, search for iatrogenic proximal margin imperfections in metal fillings.

Grade Ø: No restoration on the proximal surface.

Grade C: No iatrogenic imperfection! But proximal surface alteration observed on radiograph as a radiolucency in the enamel surface (caries, Grade D_1, D_2).

Grade 0: Restored proximal surface without visible imperfection.

Grade 1: Imperfection suspected.

Grade 2: Imperfection certain, <1.0 mm

Grade 3: Imperfection certain, >1.0 mm
   −: Surface not scored because of radiolucent filling or overlapping of teeth.

Enter your findings in the scheme below, under "Radiographically-evident Irritants." Make the entries for the maxilla above the corresponding tooth number, those for the mandible below, mesially or distally according to what surface you are scoring. Cross out missing teeth! Sketch in any bridgework present.

Radiographically-evident Irritants

18   17   16   15   14   13   12   11   21   22   23   24   25   26   27   28

48   47   46   45   44   43   42   41   31   32   33   34   35   36   37   38

Questions:

How many surfaces were scored? _____
How many of the scored surfaces exhibited imperfections of Grade

Ø _____   1 _____

C _____   2 _____

0 _____   3 _____

2. Irritants and inflammation

Determine the degree of inflammation in the papilla region using the SB Index. Probe the col region:

a) in interdental areas where neither proximal surfaces have fillings ($\emptyset$) or where they are Grade 0 filled. Surfaces which have no fillings often exhibit proximal chalky spots, however. But because the initial stage of caries involvement does not effect the morphology of the enamel surface, either radiographic D_1 or D_2 surfaces may be used in this exercise. Indicate these with a C.

b) in interdental areas with marginal imperfections of Grades 2 and 3.

With the periodontal probe, determine the maximum SBI score by probing mesial and distal areas from both oral and facial aspects. Enter these data in *red* on the chart of radiographically-evident irritants, between the numbers designating the teeth in question. Calculate the average SB Index for the P units.

	Number of radiographically evaluated proximal surfaces (N)	Average P Index
Unfilled $\emptyset$ or Grades C or O filled proximal surfaces	_____	_____
Filled proximal surfaces, Grades 2 or 3	_____	_____

3. Radiographic and clinical diagnosis of marginal irritants

Check with the explorer and with dental floss all radiographic Grade 0 and Grade 1 proximal surfaces.

	Number of radiographic Grade 0 and Grade 1 surfaces	Percent clinically perfect
	_____	_____

Instructor's signature: _____

Discussion of Exercise Results

1. Frequency of radiographically evident imperfections

A total of 446 filled and 998 unfilled proximal surfaces in 28 students were evaluated radiographically, with the following results:

All subjects had at least one suspected or definitely imperfect proximal filling. Only 50.2% of all observed proximal restorations were radiographically perfect.

	Total Number	per Subject (N = 28)
Total examined surfaces	1444	51.6
Unfilled surfaces Grade 0	998 (69.1 %)	35.6
Filled surfaces, Grades 0, 1, 2, 3	446 (30.9 %)	15.9
Grade 0 surfaces (radioraphically perfect)	224 (50.2 %)	48.0
Grade 1 surfaces (radiographically suspect)	144 (32.4 %)	5.1
Grade 2 surfaces	60 (13.4 %)	2.1
Grade 3 surfaces	18 (4.0 %)	0.64

17.4% of the proximal fillings were undoubtedly inadequate (marginal imperfections of Grades 2 and 3), but the true figure was probably higher. In fact, a combined radio-graphic-clinical study showed conclusively that 66% of all proximal fillings were not satisfactory.

These figures correspond well with those of Gilmore and Sheiham[1], who found severe overfilling (Grades 2 and 3) in 19.0% of 473 18- to 24-year-olds.

[1] Gilmore and Sheiham: Overhanging dental restorations and periodontal disease. J. Periodont. 42, 1: 1971.

See also: Renggli, H. and Regolati, B.: Gingival inflammation and plaque accumulation by well-adapted supragingival and subgingival proximal restorations. Helv. odont. Acta 16, 99; 1972.

2. Irritants and gingival inflammation

	Average no. and range of radiographically observed proximal surfaces	Average SB Index of P units
Unfilled or Grade 0 filled proximal surfaces	20.9 ± 10.2 3 − 47	0.26 ± 0.32 0 − 1
Grade 2 or 3 filled proximal surfaces	4.9 ± 3.8 1 − 15	0.71 ± 0.62 0 − 2

The degree of gingival inflammation is twice as high adjacent to unsatisfactory proximal fillings, and this could well cause the acceleration of periodontal destruction. Overhanging fillings are correlated with more severe periodontal bone loss[1]. The same is true for inadequate crown margins, as demonstrated by the following example:

a) Gold crowns and gingivitis[2]

175 newly-seated gold crowns were examined radiographically after they had been in the mouth for 5 years. The crowned teeth were compared to homologous, uncrowned teeth in the same dentitions.

Degree of inflammation of the periodontium of crowned teeth as compared to the periodontium of uncrowned teeth. Number of crowns.

Degree of inflammation after 5 years	Marginal adaptation of the crown good		inadequate		total	
less	0		0		0	
same amount	61	53 %	16	27 %	77	44 %
slightly more	44	38 %	25	42 %	69	39 %
much more	11	9 %	18	31 %	29	17 %
Totals	116	64 %	59	36 %	175	100 %

In 15% of cases, secondary cervical carious lesions were also in evidence.

[1] Odont. Rev. 20, 311; 1969.

[2] Finn. dent. J. 66, 275; 1970.

b) Gold crowns and periodontal disease[1]

387 gold crowns were checked radiographically for the quality of the proximal marginal adaptation, and for periodontal bone destruction. Results were compared to homologous teeth without marginal irritation. 83% (!) of cast gold crowns were found to be unsatisfactory; 74% of veneered crowns were unsatisfactory.

Defective proximal margins (>0.2 mm) were found in 68% of gold crowns ad in 57% of veneered crowns.

Marginal periodontal bone loss associated with poor margins, compared to uncrowned control teeth

Type of Imperfection	Degree of Imperfection	Amount of bone loss	Significance as compared to control
Overhang	<0.2 mm	0.71 mm	P<0.001
	>0.2 mm	0.66 mm	P<0.05
Undercontour	obvious	1.31 mm!	P<0.02

3. Radiographic and clinical diagnosis of marginal irritants

Number and range of examined radiographic Grade 0 and Grade 1 surfaces	Percentage of these which were clinically perfect
10.7 ± 9.0	49.6 ± 28.7
$2 - 32$	

The high art of restorative dentistry again becomes apparent in a statistical study dealing with the frequency and causes of failure of crowns and bridges[2].

Percentage frequency of failure with crowns and bridges:

During year	1	7.2%
Cumulative to end of year	2	13.5%
	3	20.4%
	7	50.7%
	11	66.0%
	15	78.2%

After only 7 years, half of all crowns and bridges require replacement. The causes of the failures are numerous and affect the function of the restorations to varying degrees.

[1] Odont. Revy 21, 337; 1970.

[2] J.A.D.A. 81, 1395; 1970.

Reasons for inadequacy of crowns and bridges[1]   N = 791

Causes of failure	Percent frequency of failure	Serviceability of the restoration, in years
Caries	36.8	11.1
Loosening of the crown	12.1	6.8
Poor margin adaptation	11.3	9.7
Severe attrition	7.4	13.1
Periodontal disease	6.8	15.5
Loosening of teeth	4.4	10.9
Loss of veneer	3.7	5.1
Cosmetic reasons	3.3	9.3
Periapical infection	2.9	5.3
Solder joint break	2.9	6.5
Other	5.5	–

The prognosis for dental restorations also depends to a great degree upon the ability of the dentist. Mistakes made by the dentist which led to failure of a filling were reported in an English statistical study[2] with the following frequencies:

Number of examined teeth: 887

Fracture of the filling	4%	Poor marginal adaptation	41%
Tooth fracture	6%	Remaining caries	2%
Inadequate retention	6%	Loss of filling due to incorrect	
Inadequate extension	25%	cavity preparation	16%

Poor marginal adaptation (marginal irritation) and inadequate extension of filling margins alone account for 66% of the failures.

We must get away from the dogmatic belief that gold restorations last longer than ones made from other materials. The maximum in vivo duration of various filling materials was found to be as follows (in years):

Gold foil	45	Bridges	15	Gold inlay	13	Acrylic crown	3
Amalgam	25	Silicate	13	Porcelain crown 12			

[1]   J.A.D.A. 81, 1395; 1970.

[2]   Brit. dent. J. 126, 172; 1969.

In this connection, it is also interesting to look at the amount of work performed by dentists. 2,593 American dentists reported their work performed on 35,793 patients[1].

Dentist's tasks per 100 persons per year

Examinations   41.8
Calculus removal   38.4
Radiographs   134.4
Fillings   106.9
Extractions   28.0 (far too many!)
Single crowns   5.7
Bridges   2.0
Full dentures   3.0
Partial dentures   2.1
Orthodontic treatment 10.0
Periodontal treatment   4.2 (far too few!)
Root canal treatment   4.6
Fluoride treatment   6.1

Conclusion Regarding Marginal Irritants

It is impossible to treat all carious lesions perfectly. On the basis of the results just presented, who could claim otherwise? All the more reason for the maxim: *Don't let the patient's dentition get to the point of needing fillings!*

Marginal Irritation:

> Miss Papilla stook naked and willing,
> Near a newly-placed amalgam filling.
> > But the margin hung over
> > Took advantage of her.
> For her, the rough passion was killing.

[1] J.A.D.A. 81, 25; 1970.

Epidemiology of Periodontal Disease

Instruction Sheet

X-1: Epidemiology of the periodontal diseases

Material

Student: periodontal probe, mouth mirror

Instructor: radiographic surveys of periodontal patients

In a dental school situation, it is usually not very beneficial to have students investigate periodontal disease epidemiology by examining each other, because in young dental students one generally detects only gingivitis or the very earliest manifestations of periodontal disease. Ideally, several clinic patients with moderate to severe periodontal disease may be asked to be present during this Exercise so that students may observe first hand the clinical picture of periodontal destruction. However, if this is not possible, there are usually (and unfortunately!) at least a few students who exhibit obvious periodontal destruction. It is recommended that the periodontal indices be demonstrated on these students. If necessary, the material of this exercise can be presented didactically alone, following Exercise VIII.

Epidemiology of Periodontal Diseases

Included here is an overview of the epidemiological diagnosis of periodontal disease. The various periodontal indices are explained fully. Even though students may not have the opportunity to practice them, such knowledge is absolutely necessary if the dentist is to understand the significance of what he reads in the literature.

Some frightening periodontal disease statistics:

1/3 of all adults have severe periodontal disease.
1/10 of all adults lose their teeth exclusively because of periodontal disease.

Periodontal disease is surffered by:

2/3 of all young adults
4/5 of "middle-aged" adults
9/10 of all people over 65.

After age 35, periodontal disease is the primary cause of tooth loss. After age 40, two-thirds of all teeth lost are lost due to periodontal disease. After the age of 15, periodontal disease is reponsible for 50% of tooth loss, while dental caries accounts for 3,7%.

Periodontal indices are of practical value only in epidemiological studies and not in incidence investigations.

Indices[1] are used:

- to determine the frequences, and the severity of the disease in certain groups of people in a population or within age groups. This information may reveal to what degree a specific treatment is necessary.

- to compare the frequences and severity in different groups in a population. By comparing such information with other data concerning circumstances or conditions which accompany the disease, etiological factors may become known.

- to estimate the success of treatment methods in altering the usual further manifestations of the disease in several groups of a population.

[1] Literature covering periodontal indices: Summary in Schweiz. Mschr. Zahnheilk. 74, 7; 1964.

The Periodontal Index (PI)

The "Periodontal Index" of Russell[1] is used in most epidemiological studies.

This index assesses destructive marginal periodontitis and is scored on the assumption that periodontal disease progresses in the following sequence: gingival inflammation → pocket formation → bone loss → decreased function (increased tooth mobility) → tooth loss.

Method

Every tooth present in each subject is scored according to the following system:

0 = No alterations.

1 = Slight gingivitis, areas of inflammation present on the gingival margin, but not continuous around the tooth. Example: papillitis.

2 = Severe gingivitis. Inflammation all around the tooth. No true pockets.

4 = Irregular early resorptions of the alveolar ridge, visible in the radiograph (However, the PI is generally performed without the use of x-rays).

6 = Severe gingivitis plus true pocket formation. Tooth mobility still normal; tooth still functional. (On the radiograph, horizontal bone loss evident around the entire tooth and extending as far as half way to the apex.)

8 = Severe gingivitis + pocket formation + advanced destruction and loss of tooth function. Tooth loosening coupled with axial mobility. Dull sound upon percussion. (Radiographic evidence of advanced bone loss involving more than half the root length. Bony pockets. Widened periodontal ligament space.)

Calculation of the Periodontal Index: Sum all tooth scores and divide by the number of teeth examined. The Periodontal Index underestimates the actual conditions, especially if teeth have already been lost due to periodontal disease. Consider, for example, the following clinical situation:

Subject with these teeth still present

| 13 | 12 | 11 | | 21 | 22 | 23 | |
| 43 | 42 | 41 | | 31 | 32 | 33 | with an average PI of $\bar{x} = 1.0$. |

Don't you think this PI is too low if all posterior teeth had to be extracted 5 years ago because of deep periodontal pockets?

The PI gives primarily differences in advanced disease and when most of the teeth are still present. The index is not very sensitive to early disease. Since all teeth are scored, it also requires considerable time.

[1] J. dent. Res. 35, 350; 1956.

Example of an epidemiological investigation[1] (simplified figures)

| | Periodontal Index | |
	20-yr-olds	50-yr-olds
Alaska	0.45	1.0
Ethiopia	0.6	2.0
Lebanon	0.35	4.0
Thailand	0.4	5.0

Correlations were calculated from PI and OHI data obtained in Lebanon and Vietnam. r = 0.96 for the correlation between age, PI and OHI. An exact analysis shows that the periodontal condition is 36 to 42% age-dependent and 51 to 56% dependent upon the degree of oral cleanliness (OHI).

Average PI of people in India (W.H.O. study)

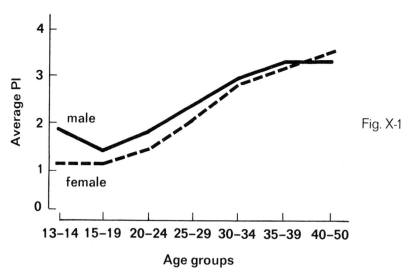

Fig. X-1

The Periodontal Disease Index (Ramfjord)

Because the PI underestimates the actual condition with regard to periodontal de-struction, Ramfjord[2] developed the "Periodontal Disease Index" (PDI). Only six teeth are scored: 16, 21, 24 and 44, 41, 36. The PDI represents a combination of the SBI, recession index and a "pocket PI index."

Grades 1–3 indicate the severity of gingivitis (G).

[1] J. dent. Res. 42, 233; 1963.
[2] J. Periodont. 30, 51; 1959.

Grades 4–6 indicate periodontal destruction (bone loss), independent of the severity of gingivitis. Grades 4–6 may indicate gingival recession and/or pocket depth.

Method

Degree of gingivitis:

0 = healthy

1 = mild gingivitis affecting only a part of the periodontium, e. g., only papilla involved.

2 = mild gingivitis, extending around the entire tooth (P+M).

3 = severe gingivitis, with intense reddening, heavy bleeding, ulceration and swelling.

Periodontal destruction

Bone loss is measured from the cementoenamel junction (CEJ). This score may represent pure recession, or pocketing alone, or a combination of both these phenomena. Measurements are made in millimeters on 4 surfaces of each tooth.

Two possible situations:

1) The gingival margin (GM) is located upon enamel

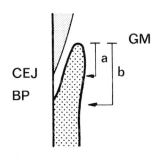

a   = distance from GM to CEJ

b   = GM to BP (base of pocket)

b–a = periodontal destruction

2) Gingival margin is located upon root cementum

c   = CEJ to GM (expressed as a negative number)

d   = CEJ to BP

c + d   = periodontal destruction

Fig. X-2

The greatest loss (b−a, or d) in millimeters, found among the four tooth surfaces is transposed into grades, according to its severity.

Loss up to and including 3 mm   = Grade 4
Loss from 3–6 mm   = Grade 5
Loss over 6 mm   = Grade 6

Here are some examples of practical application of the PD index. The 4 teeth depicted in Fig. X-3 are shown with the various PDI scores which were found clinically. A brief explanation of these scores appears at the left.

Interpretation

Gingival margin is located every-where upon enamel. Deepest loss is 4 minus 1 = 3 mm

Thus: Grade 4

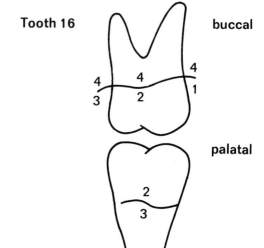

Tooth 16   buccal

palatal

Interpretation

Buccally, the gingival margin is located upon the root surface (−2 = 2 mm recession). Deep-est loss on the buccal = 5 mm.

Thus: Grade 5

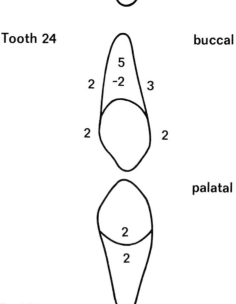

Tooth 24   buccal

palatal

Fig. X-3

If no periodontal destruction is present, the gingivitis score (anywhere from 1 to 3) is entered. The sum of the periodontal destruction grades or the gingivitis grades, devided by the number of teeth scored (6) gives the total destruction value. One problem is that the CEJ is often difficult to locate.

In addition to gingivitis, the Ramfjord system evaluates the following:

Calculus (C)
0 = none
1 = supragingival, approx. 1 mm thick at the gingival margin
2 = moderate supra- and/or subgingival calculus
3 = abundant supra- and subgingival calculus

Attrition (A)
0 = none
1 = only in enamel
2 = into the dentin on chewing surfaces
3 = extreme; occlusal surfaces exhibit reverse contours; cusps are hollowed out like throughs

Tooth mobility (M)
0 = normal, teeth are firm
1 = slightly more than normal
2 = more evident, but no loss of tooth function
3 = extreme, total loss of function of the tooth

Diastemata (D)
0 = none
1 = 1 mm separation
2 = 2−3 mm separation
3 = more than 3 mm separation

Plaque (P)
0 = none
1 = spots of plaque on some interdental and gingival areas
2 = plaque in all interdental areas
3 = plaque in all interdental areas; more than half of each tooth surface found covered with plaque after use of disclosing agent

The PDI gingivitis-periodontal destruction index also requires considerable time, because 6 x 4 surfaces must be evaluated. In field studies, it is hardly more efficient than the PI, but somewhat more sensitive. The PDI, too, underestimates the true situation.

In Switzerland, in 1972, Curilović et al.[1] used the PDI for the first time on a diverse group of military recruits. Relatively favorable periodontal conditions were reported, in comparison to data from Ramfjord's investigations. In more than half the recruits, the PDI varied between Grades 3.1 and 4.0. 96% exhibited gingivitis and not one recruit had a plaque-free dentition. On the average, calculus was not frequently detected.

[1] Curilović, Z., Renggli, H. H., Saxer, U. P., Germann, M. A.: Parodontalzustand bei einer Gruppe von Schweizer Rekruten. Schweiz. Mschr. Zahnheilk. 82, 437; 1972.

The clinically measurable sulcus depth was found to range from 1.0 to 2.5 mm. Pockets of depth greater than 3 mm were seldom encountered. Recession of the gingiva to below the CEJ was almost never observed. Tooth mobility was normal in 99% of the recruits. On the other hand, almost all recruits had attrition facets of various degrees of severity.

PDI, calculus and plaque indices in young Indians[1]

Age	N	PDI	Calculus	Plaque
11	343	1.33	0.91	1.73
13	255	1.45	1.20	1.65
15	189	1.53	1.23	1.54
17	40	1.42	1.33	1.55

Comparison of PI and PDI

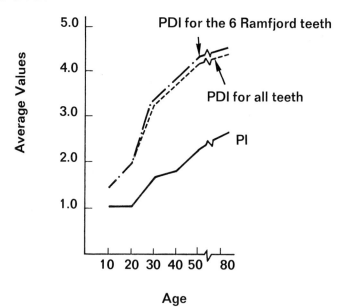

Fig. X-4

[1] Ramfjord, S. P.: The periodontal status of boys 11 to 17-years-old in Bombay, India. J. Periodont. 32, 237; 1961.

The Periodontal Disease Rate Index[1] (PDR)

The PDR is quick, simple and certain. For each subject, the number of periodontally diseased teeth is determined as a percentage of the total number of teeth present.

A tooth is considered to be periodontally diseased if at least one of the following four criteria are met:

a) there is gingivitis all around the tooth, with or without hypertrophy or necrosis of the gingiva.

b) there is a periodontal pocket 3 mm deep.

c) tooth mobility of 1 mm can be detected.

d) there is radiographic evidence of 3 mm bone loss.

Thus, in a subject with 7 periodontally diseased and 5 periodontally healthy teeth,

$$PDR = \frac{7}{(7 + 5)} = 0.58$$

There is a rather close correlation between the PDR and the PI of Russell.

[1] Sandler, Stahl: JADA 58, 93; 1959

Additional literature

Greene, J. C.: Epidemiology and indexing of periodontal disease. J. Periodont. 30, 133; 1959.

Lilienthal, B., Amerana, V., Gregory, G.: A comparison of a modified periodontal scoring system with Russell's periodontal index. Arch. oral Biol. 9, 575; 1964.

Glavind, L., Löe, H.: Errors in the clinical assessment of periodontal destruction. J. periodont. Res. 2, 180; 1967.

Roy, E. J., Clemmer, B. A.: Reproducibility of periodontal indices. US Navy Med. 59, 41; 1972.

Hassell, T. M., Germann, M. A., Saxer, U. P.: Periodontal probing: Interinvestigator discrepancies and correlations between probing force and recorded depth. Helv. odont. Acta 17, 38; 1973.

Enamel Defects

Instruction Sheet

XI-1: Enamel opacities

XI-2: Systemic enamel hypoplasia

XI-3: Tetracycline staining of the teeth

XI-4: Mottled enamel

Exercise Sheet

XI-4: Measurement of enamel opacities

Results Sheet

XI-4: Measurement of enamel opacities

Material

Student: mouth mirror, explorer, cotton pliers

Instructor: color rings, UV light

Program

1. Discussion of results from Exercise X

2. Introduction to today's topic

3. Exercises

Enamel Opacities

Synonyms: Internal enamel hypoplasia
              Opaque enamel spots
              Idiopathic enamel spots

Enamel opacities are acquired preeruptively. They are opaque-white, sometimes yellowish, sharply demarcated spots on the morphologically intact, smooth enamel surface. These are single spots, randomly scattered over the enamel surface. Enamel opacities may be found on one or several permanent teeth, or in primary tooth enamel which was formed postnatally. They are frequently seen on the incisal third of anterior teeth, and on the cusp tips of premolars and molars. Enamel opacities are more pronounced on labial surfaces as opposed to lingual surfaces. The spots are visible because of altered light reflectance.

At the electron microscopic level, enamel opacities are seen to be the result of disorientation of the apatite crystals at the periphery of the enamel rod. In addition to microspaces, enlarged crystals may also be present.

The nitrogen content of the spots is higher. They are less radiopaque, but this is observable only on *micro*-radiographs!

The differential diagnosis should include:

1. Mottled enamel (dental fluorosis)

2. Chalky spot: posteruptive initial carious lesion at typical predilection sites on
                the crown.

3. Systemically induced hypoplasia

4. Tetracycline staining of the tooth

Frequency of enamel opacities on permanent teeth

In six studies including a total of 4,430 children (12 to 21-years-old), enamel opacities were found in 21.8 to 35.9% (mean 28%) of cases. They were more frequently observed in the maxilla than in the mandible, especially on teeth 11 and 21!

Cause:

An enamel opacity is the result of a local, non-systemic disturbance of enamel formation. Perhaps trauma to the deciduous precursor is one cause of opacity in the permanent tooth. This whole area of enamel opacities has not been comprehensively researched.

Anti-fluoridationists again and again attribute the benign and frequently observed enamel opacities to fluoride treatments and describe them as examples of mottled enamel. For this reason, it is very important to differentiate simple enamel opacities from mottled enamel, as well as from systemic hypoplasia and tetracycline staining. Investigations of students revealed enamel opacities at a frequency of 60%. In students with enamel opacities, 4 to 6 teeth were generally affected.

It is obvious that data concerning the frequency of occurrence of enamel opacities are quite dependent upon the definition of opacity. A quick glance at the anterior teeth is not sufficient for the detection of small opacities which are not aesthetically bothersome. Such spots are, in reality, color alterations. An interesting article about color diagnosis in dentistry was published by Sproull[1].

[1] Sproull, R. C.: Color matching in dentistry. Part I. The three-dimensional nature of color. J. Prosth. Dent. 29, 416–424; 1973. Part II. Practical applications of the organization of color. J. Prosth. Dent. 29, 556–566; 1973.

Systemic Enamel Hypoplasia

Systemic enamel hypoplasia results from a disturbance of the general metabolism (e. g., avitaminosis, severe disease states) which occurs during tooth development. It is manifested as symmetrical enamel alterations involving homologous teeth. Hypoplasias of this type are often combined with macroscopic enamel defects such as pits, grooves and cracks which may become stained after tooth eruption.

The distribution of enamel hypoplasias in the dentition and on the various tooth crowns corresponds to the chronology of tooth crown development (see chart, page 183). 65% of systemic enamel hypoplasias occur during the first 10 months of life (teeth 12 and 22 develop only after this time). The mesial cusps of the first permanent molars develop prenatally.

The enamel changes are associated with alterations in the dentin (interglobular dentin).

The primary disturbance probably takes place during matrix development by the ameloblasts and/or odontoblasts. This may occur prenatally (seldom), neonatally and/or postnatally.

Children born prematurely (ca. 2.5 kg birth weight) often have neonatal enamel defects. These usually are located at the gingival third of primary teeth 51 and 61. Hypoplasias of this type can lead to melanodontia, a severe carious lesion in the cervical region of deciduous incisors. Melanodontia frequently becomes evident when a child is repeatedly given a sugar-coated rubber pacifier to suck.

Epidemiology

Systemic enamel hypoplasia was much more frequently observed in the past than it is today (rickets prevention!). In fact, "rickets hypoplasia" was once a common term.

Frequency of systemic enamel hypoplasia on permanent teeth in Sweden:

1937/8	14–15 yrs.	N = 2,000	20.0 %
1944	9–14 yrs.	N = 2,586	14.6 %
1954	12–28 yrs.	N = 64	3.1 %

The frequency in the primary dentition in 1958 in Sweden was 2%, especially in deciduous cuspids and molars.

Chronology of Development of Deciduous and Permanent Teeth[1]

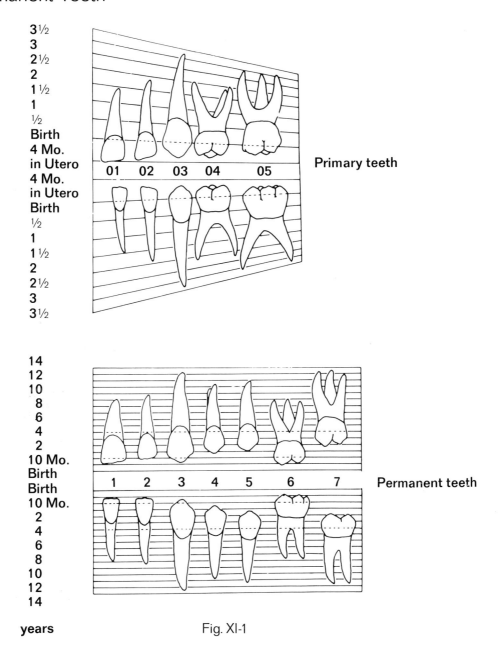

Fig. XI-1

[1] Massler, Schour and Poncher. In: Pindborg, J. J.: Pathology of the Dental Hard Tissues. Munksgaard, Copenhagen, 1970.

Age in years of permanent teeth at termination of Crown development and at Eruption into the oral cavity (means).

Tooth type		Termination of crown development		Clinical eruption	
		male	female	male	female
Central incisor	max.	3.3	3.3	6.9	6.7
	mand.	–	–	6.3	6.2
Lateral incisor	max.	4.6	4.4	8.3	7.8
	mand.	3.3	–	7.3	6.8
Cuspid	max.	4.6	4.5	12.1	10.6
	mand.	4.3	4.1	10.2	9.6
First bicuspid	max.	6.8	6.3	10.2	9.6
	mand.	5.9	5.4	10.3	9.6
Second bicuspid	max.	7.1	6.6	11.4	10.2
	mand.	7.0	6.4	11.1	10.1
First molar	max.	3.6	3.5	6.4	6.4
	mand.	3.5	3.5	6.3	6.3
Second molar	max.	7.3	6.9	12.8	12.4
	mand.	7.4	7.0	.12.2	11.4
Third molar	max.	13.2	12.8	–	–
	mand.	13.7	13.3	–	–

These results were compiled by orthopantomographic analysis of 1,162 Finnish children (1965–1968)[1].

[1] Kaarina Haavikko: The formation and the alveolar and clinical eruption of the permanent teeth. Finn. dent. J. 66, 103–170; 1970.

Tetracycline Staining of the Teeth

The stains caused by tetracycline are gray-yellowish, yellowish or dark brown discolorations of the tooth crown, especially in the deciduous dentition. Teeth so stained fluoresce a light yellow color when viewed under an UV light[1]. Tetracycline which is administered systemically (e. g., for the treatment of cystic fibrosis) is incorporated into the tooth substance during tooth development, and especially into the dentin along the lines of growth. Less deposition occurs in the enamel. The discoloration is often observed in combination with hypoplastic enamel defects, but scientists are still not sure whether such hypoplastic defects are caused by the tetracycline *per se*, or by the underlying systemic disease being treated with the drug.

Mechanism of staining

It is probable that the tetracycline induces calcium chelation, thereby inhibiting the nucleation of apatite. It also hinders crystal growth and the transformation of octa-calcium phosphate into apatite.

A single dose of tetracycline can lead to staining of the teeth. The critical "staining period" is primarily during the phase of enamel-dentin development at the cervical third of the tooth. A dose of 20 mg/kg body weight is sufficient for staining. Fortunately, the staining may decrease with time.

The primary teeth will be stained yellow if tetracycline is administered up to the 9th month of life. Taking the drug after this time will also lead to obvious staining of some permanent teeth. The first permanent molar may be stained if the drug is taken after the sixth month of life. Tetracycline crosses the placenta. Therefore, expectant mothers should not take this drug after the 29th week (7th month) of pregnancy!

The frequency of tetracycline staining is, of course, dependent upon pediatric treatment methods and upon the subjects selected for examination. In a total of 1,724 healthy 5 to 9-year-old schoolchildren, 2.3% had tetracycline stains. In Australia, 3.4% of 4,690 four to 17-year-old schoolchildren were affected, 0.5% severely[2]. The incidence of tetracycline staining was 29% among 63 pediatric patients three to 8-years-old[3].

There are several different types of tetracycline*. The amount of yellow staining they can produce diminishes in the following order:

[1] Hefferren, J. J. et al.: Use of ultraviolet illumination in oral diagnosis. JADA 82, 1353; 1971.

[2] Med. J. Aust. 1, 1286; 1969.

[3] J. dent. child. 37, 117; 1970.

* Translator's note: Some of the drugs listed here are available in Switzerland, but not necessarily in many other countries. The spellings are as in the German original, and all are included for the sake of completeness. There are undoubtedly other brands of tetracycline on the world market.

Ledermycin = Demecyclin = Dimethylchortetracycline. This drug produces the most severe staining.

Tetralysol = tetracycline methylenelysine

Achromycin (the name is incorrect!) = Diocyclin, Hostacyclin, Mephacyclin, Supramycin, Triphacyclin. All of these products are tetracycline hydrochlorides.

Aureomycin = chlortetracycline-HCl. This drug produces a stain which is more grayish-brown.

Terramycin = oxytetracycline

Rondomycin = Metacyclin = methylenehydroxytetracycline

Vibramycin = Doxycyclin = deoxyhydroxytetracycline. This drug causes less severe staining.

Mottled Enamel

(Dental fluorosis)

Mottled enamel appears as enamel alterations resulting from toxic damage to the amelo-blasts by fluoride during enamel development. During the diagnosis, it is very important to clarify whether the enamel alterations resulted from a lengthly intake of excessive fluoride (e. g., through living up to the age of 8 in an area where the water supply had >1.5 ppm F) or came about merely because of a short-term (days or weeks) fluoride intoxication.

The distribution of the mottling is symmetrical, and corresponds to the chronology of enamel development. Labial tooth surfaces are more severely affected as a rule than are oral surfaces. Mandibular anterior teeth generally exhibit less pronounced mottling than do maxillary anterior teeth.

Whenever you suspect mottling, you should take a complete and detailed history, using a questionnaire for enamel opacities (see pp. 188–192).

Primary teeth indicated for extraction or ones which the patient may have kept after their exfoliation can be extremely valuable. The determination of an increased F content in peripheral dentin of the tooth crown, in the enamel and in the urine[1] usually confirms the diagnosis of dental fluorosis. Enamel formed before birth is practically never mottled because of the relative placental barrier to the passage of fluoride. Mottling of the enamel of permanent teeth cannot occur, of course, after the end of crown development (amelogenesis).

---

[1] Regolati, B., Hotz, P.: Die Zahnfluorose. Eine Erläuterung anhand von 3 klinischen Fällen. Schweiz. Mschr. Zahnheilk. 83, 576; 1973.

Questionnaire Concerning Dental Fluorosis

The child's history of exposure to fluoride should be taken during conversation with the mother.

Laste name: _____   Address: _____

First name: _____   _____

Date of birth: _____   _____

Siblings: _____   Ages: _____

_____   _____

_____   _____

_____   _____

_____   _____

Domicile: as a baby _____   F ppm in drinking water _____

later _____   _____

_____   _____

_____   _____

Diet History

How long was the child breast fed? 0, 1, 2, 3, 4, 5, 6, 7, 8, 9 months

Did the child receive milk or fruit juice in such amounts that the intake of communal drinking water was considerably less in comparison to a child who received drinks prepared by mixing powders with tap water?

                                    YES   NO
                                  [   ]   [   ]

If yes: At what age was the intake of water from the communal water supply relatively low?

                                    ½, 1, 2, 3, 4, 5-years-old

Does your family drink a great deal of black tea?

    If so, at what age did the child begin drinking the tea?   _____

    How much per day   _____

Does the child eat sardines or other sea fish frequently?

                                  [   ]   [   ]

If so, at what age did the child begin to like eating sardines or sea fish? _____

	YES	NO
Are they eaten less than once per week?	☐	☐
Once per week?	☐	☐
More than once per week?	☐	☐

Is bottled mineral water drunk regularly in the home?   ☐ ☐

Brand name? _____

If yes: At what age did the child begin to drink it regularly? _____

Do you use fluoridated cooking salt?*   ☐ ☐

Since what year?   19_____

Did the child like to eat heavily salted foods at age

2–5 years?	☐	☐
5–8 years?	☐	☐

Was the child often thirsty and did he therefore require a high intake of liquids?

2–5 years?	☐	☐
5–8 years?	☐	☐

Did the child receive bone meal preparations?   ☐ ☐

Which one? _____

At what age? _____

At what age was toothbrushing begun?
2, 3, 4, 5, 6-years-old

Was a fluoride-containing dentifrice used?   ☐ ☐
Which one? _____

* Translator's note: The use of fluoridated cooking salt has been widespread in Switzerland since before 1962.

Was the fluoride dentifrice used at age

3–5 years: once per day   ☐   ☐

                                     twice per day   ☐   ☐

5–8 years: once per day   ☐   ☐

                                     twice per day   ☐   ☐

When did you begin to give your child fluoride tablets daily
at home?

	YES	NO	How many tablets?	What brand?
Pregnancy?	☐	☐	_____	_____
1st year of life?	☐	☐	_____	_____
1 – 3 years?	☐	☐	_____	_____
3 – 5 years?	☐	☐	_____	_____
5 – 8 years?	☐	☐	_____	_____

Did the child receive fluoride tablets in kindergarten? at school?

	YES	NO	How many tablets?	What brand?
age 4	☐	☐	_____	_____
age 5	☐	☐	_____	_____
age 6	☐	☐	_____	_____
age 7	☐	☐	_____	_____

Have you, at home, performed any other types of fluoridation, for example adding
fluoride to milk? Have you used any special fluoride preparations other than F-tooth-
pastes?

	YES	NO
1–3 years?	☐	☐
3–5 years?	☐	☐
5–8 years?	☐	☐

In kindergarten or at school, did the child receive any other fluoride applications?

	YES	NO
Fluoride solutions?	☐	☐
Fluoride gels?	☐	☐
Fluorides pastes?	☐	☐

Clinical findings in mottling

Which primary teeth are still present in the mouth? (circle if present)

55 54 53 52 51   61 62 63 64 65

85 84 83 82 81   71 72 73 74 75

Chart of opacities (see example at right)

White opacities:

Sketch in the outline of these

Yellow-brown opacities:

Make dots to indicate these

Brown opacities:

Fill these in solidly

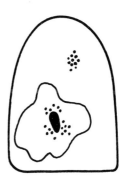

facial

Maxilla

Mandible

occlusal

Maxilla

Mandible

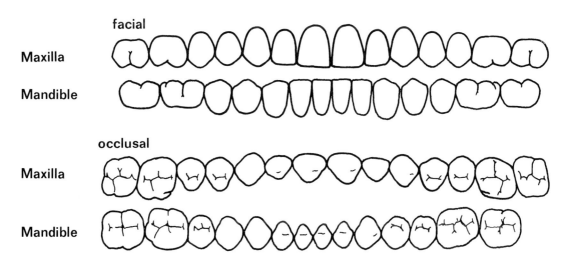

Fig. X-2

Hypoplastic defects

Are any present? If so, on which teeth?
(circle in scheme below)

| 18 | 17 | 16 | 15 | 14 | 13 | 12 | 11 | | 21 | 22 | 23 | 24 | 25 | 26 | 27 | 28 |
| 48 | 47 | 46 | 45 | 44 | 43 | 42 | 41 | | 31 | 32 | 33 | 34 | 35 | 36 | 37 | 38 |

Were color photographs taken?   Date: _____

24-hour urine collection for F measurement? Date: _____

Enamel biopsy?   Date: _____

Dentin biopsy?   Where? _____

                                                                    Date: _____

Additional observations or comments:

Date: _____ Examining dentist: _____

P.S.

When possible, siblings and even the parents should also be examined. This may help to establish the cause of the opacities.

Measurement of Enamel Opacities

1. Determine the color of the upper incisor teeth using the color ring:

a) in daylight,

b) in artificial light.

2. Using the color ring in daylight, determine the color of the

a) mandibular incisors,

b) mandibular canines.

3. On the facial surfaces only of all teeth, look for

a) Enamel opacities (EO): white or yellowish-brown spots not associated with any alteration of the enamel surface contour. Don't mistake these for chalky spots (caries)!

b) Enamel defects (ED): external enamel hypoplasias, alterations in the enamel surface contour.

Enter EO and ED on the chart (p. 191); estimate in square millimeters the size of these opacities or defects.

Example

EO are depicted as dots. Enter mm² estimate beneath the tooth diagram, as shown.

ED are depicted as black areas. Circle the mm² estimate.

Tooth number	11	21	22	23

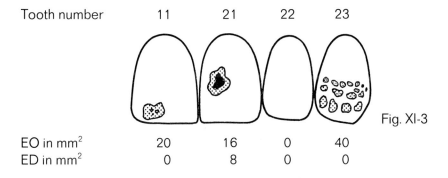

Fig. XI-3

	11	21	22	23
EO in mm²	20	16	0	40
ED in mm²	0	8	0	0

Discussion of Exercise Results

Enamel opacities (EO), enamel defects (ED)

In 22 students examined, 14 exhibited EO and 10 had discrete ED on the facial surfaces of the entire dentition. (Thus, frequency per dentition = 65% for EO and 45% for ED.) The causes of these EO and ED appeared to be local in nature in 44%, of systemic origin in 22%, and idiopathic in 34%.

Students with EO had an average of 4.0 teeth involved. Those with ED had 2.5 teeth involved.

It is obvious, therefore, that enamel opacities are a common finding.

Chewing Function and Plaque, Oral Sugar Clearance and Saliva

Instruction Sheets

XII-1: Self-cleansing of the dentition

XII-2: Oral sugar clearance

XII-3: Saliva flow rate

Exercise and Data Sheets

XII-1: Measurement of self-cleansing of the dentition

XII-2: Determination of oral sugar clearance

XII-3: Measurement of saliva flow rate

Results Sheets

XII-1: Self-cleansing of the dentition

XII-2: Oral sugar clearance

XII-3: Discussion of results

Material

Student: clinic kit, colored pencils, stopwatch. During the 2 to 3 days before this exercise is scheduled, *No Oral Hygiene* should be performed on the lingual and palatal surfaces of the teeth.

Instructor: pH indicator paper, TES-tape. Weighed measuring vessels. Coca-Cola, peanuts, carrots, lemons, apples and chewing gum.

Program

1. Discussion of results from Exercise XI, "Enamel Defects"

2. Introduction to today's topic

3. Exercises

Abbreviations

Chewing function: CF   Oral sugar clearance: OSC

Self-cleansing: SC   Saliva flow rate: SFR

Self-Cleansing of the Dentition

Do you think the dentition is actively cleaned by the chewing of hard-consistency foodstuffs? Is plaque removed? Does chewing gum clean the teeth?

The influence of self-cleansing upon caries and gingivitis was studied in England[1]; 155 children, aged 4 to 9 years, received fresh carrots as "dessert" after lunch for two years. The results were compared to those of non-carrot-eaters from the same area.

Results

1. The incidence of carious defects of Grade 3 was not influenced.

2. The degree of plaque accumulation was the same in all age groups of both carrot-eaters and non-carrot-eaters.

3. A reduction in gingivitis was not significant.

The percentage frequency of children "without severe gingivitis" is given below:

Age in years	Children "without severe gingivitis"	
	Carrots	No carrots
4 – 5	71.7	66.3
6 – 7	50.0	50.0
8 – 9	45.2	35.0 (N.S.)*

It appears that there is a tendency toward less gingival inflammation in carrot-eaters. But the observed difference could be attributed purely to chance!

[1] Brit. dent. J. 128, 535; 1970.   * N.S. = not significant.

Measurement of Self-Cleansing of the Dentition

Subject: _____

Age: _____

Examiner: _____

Date: _____

Objective:

To determine if hard-consistency foodstuffs (carrots, apples, peanuts etc.) or chewing gum have any plaque-removal efficacy. (Participants in this exercise must avoid oral hygiene procedures during the 2 to 3 days prior to this exercise. Students should be so informed at the previous class session.)

Procedure

Stain the plaque on the left side of the mouth. With a black pencil, sketch on the Figure below the exact outline of the plaque on the *lingual* (!) surfaces, taking care to keep the proportions in perspective. Then have the subject chew primarily on the left side, for 5 minutes or longer. Again stain the plaque, and sketch in the plaque outline on the same diagram, this time using a colored pencil. To make the picture more dramatic, color in the area where plaque was removed.

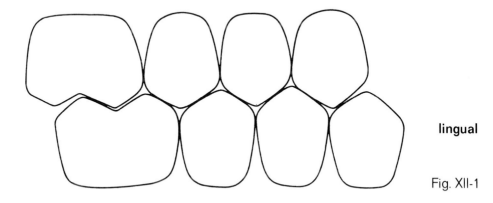

lingual

Fig. XII-1

1. What was chewed? _____ How long? _____

2. The extent of plaque removal (degree of self-cleansing) should be estimated. To what percent was plaque removed? Circle one of percentages given:

0%   10%   20%   30%   40%   50%   60%   70%   80%   90%   100%

Instructor's signature: _____

Self-Cleansing of the Dentition

Despite the chewing of hard consistency foods for an average of five minutes, plaque reduction was only $10.5 \pm 12.2\%$ (range $= 0$ to 50%), as measured in 19 subjects. Subjects who chewed chewing gum did not fare better. Self-cleansing under normal daily conditions is surely less than that evident under the ideal situation presented here. Thus, it is highly doubtful that plaque is removed from the teeth by this means. But it *is* possible that thick plaque is rendered thinner by the removal of materia alba. This possibility could not be measured through our exercise procedures. How could it be measured?

In any case, the results do not lead to the conclusion that hard, vigorous chewing is "unhealthy." On the contrary, vigorous chewing enhances the state of health of the periodontal structures. Long term hyperfunction decreases tooth mobility.

Self-Cleansing:

> A health food fanatic once said:
> "I eat only hard, dark bread.
> I chew the tough crust
> With a ravenous lust.
> Toothbrushing? ... This do I instead"!

Oral Sugar Clearance

The term "oral clearance" means the time it takes for the disappearance of a substance, e. g., sugar, fluoride etc., which has been introduced into the oral cavity.

Quantitatively, there are several ways to express the oral clearance:

Half life:

The time which passes until the maximum concentration of the substance introduced into the mouth has dropped to 50% of the original concentration (t ½).

Defined minimal concentration:

The time (S_1) which is required until a defined minimal concentration of the substance is achieved. For example, 100 mg% for glucose, or with a certain technique until glucose is no longer detectable.

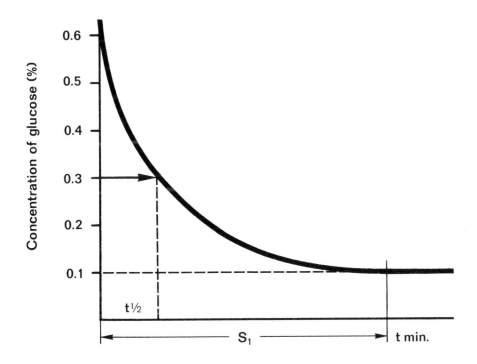

Fig. XII-2

Caries incidence is clearly dependent upon the amount of fermentable carbohydrates in the oral fluid. The quicker a substance disappears from the oral cavity, the less cariogenic it will be.

Principle

Glucose can be demonstrated in the oral fluid using TES-tape (an enzymatic method of determination). The TES-tape strips soak up the oral fluid to be tested, whereupon a chemical reaction takes place between any glucose present and the reagents impregnated in the tape.

The yellow "paper strips" (TES-tape strips) contain glucose oxidase, peroxidase and a chromogenic substance (DIH_2), which is yellow. The reactions which occur are:

I. glucose + H_2O + O_2 + *glucose oxidase* → H_2O_2 + gluconic acid.

II. H_2O_2 + DIH_2 + peroxidase → 2 H_2O + DT (0-Dianisidin-HCl, green).

The reaction requires at least one minute for maximum green coloration of the TES-tape. If the strip remains yellow, no more glucose is present in the oral fluid sampled. TES-tape reacts *only* with glucose, not with sucrose (*glucose* oxidase!)

The test strips can be used to sample the oral fluid in different regions of the oral cavity. The sugar clearance in the vestibular fold of the maxilla is different than that on the tongue or on the floor of the mouth.

Determination of the Oral Sugar Clearance

Subject (A): _____

Age: _____

Examiner (B): _____

Date: _____

Subject A drinks one glass of Coca-Cola in leisurely fashion. This soft drink contains 10% carbohydrate, about $\frac{1}{5}$ of which is glucose. Start the stopwatch immediately after the entire glass has been consumed.

Examiner B, using TES-tape, determines the time which passes before glucose completely disappears from the oral fluid:

a) on the floor of the mouth
b) in the maxillary vestibule
c) on the dorsum of the tongue.

With good organization, all three areas may be determined simultaneously.

Glucose clearance time in minutes:

a) floor of the mouth _____

b) vestibulum _____

c) tongue dorsum _____

Where do you find glucose for the longest time?

Laterally in the vestibule?   anteriorly?

Dorsum of the tongue?   or where?_____   Time:_____

Instructor's signature: _____

Oral Sugar Clearance

In an exercise involving the 18 subjects in the winter semester of 1972, the following clearance times were found:

Lateral vestibule (maxilla) (N = 9)	10.4 ± 4.9 min
Dorsum of tongue (N = 8)	8.6 ± 2.5 min

In a 1971 exercise, the results were quite similar:

Vestibulum (N = 11)	10.2 ± 3.4 min
Tongue dorsum (N = 6)	7.3 ± 3.0 min

Even though only 1/5 of the total carbohydrate content of Coca-Cola was measured (glucose), the disappearance of this cariogenic substance is nonetheless remarkably rapid.

In "normal" consumption, Coca-Cola would hardly be considered cariogenic, because of the rapid elimination of sugar from the oral cavity. But in animal caries studies, Coca-Cola is found to be one of the most cariogenic of liquids, because rats drink Coca-Cola almost constantly, day and night[1].

Sweetness and Caries

Prolonged sugar clearance time plays a most definite role in small children, as demonstrated by the following example:

Caries prevalence in 1 to 4-year-olds

601 small children were included in this study[2], which was performed in southern England in 1966–1968.

Age in months	N	Caries-free	% with rampant caries	def (Grades 3, 4)
12 – 23	172	98	0.6	0.04
24 – 35	173	82	10	0.76
36 – 47	146	64	10	1.41
48 – 60	110	42	15	3.07

[1] Helv. odont. Acta 8, 82; 1972.

[2] Winter et al.: Brit. dent. J. 130, 271; 1971.

This study considered only fully developed, readily detected large defects ($D_{3,4}$). The def for initial and advanced lesions taken together (D_{1-4}) would probably be at least twice as high. Compare these data with those from Exercise V.

It appears that this high caries prevalence is correlated with the sugar clearance: In the first place, it can be shown that caries incidence in England very generally is dependent upon socioeconomic circumstances.

Dependence of Caries Incidence on Socioeconomic Conditions

	Children N	Caries-free %	With rampant caries, %
Parents with high income	222	83	4
Parents with low income	81	56	17

When the data are analyzed with respect to caries prevalence, and in relation to breast- or bottle-feeding of infants, illness during pregnancy, premature births, childhood diseases, use of pacifiers etc., one readily finds that 12% of the children were breast-fed only, while 49% were bottle-fed only. The remaining 39% received both breast and bottle nourishment. The more natural form of nourishment (breast feeding) prevailed twice as frequently within the higher socioeconomic groups as it did among those who were socially disadvantaged. Children with caries were breast-fed for an average of 3.8 months; whereas those without caries were breast-fed for an average of 4.9 months.

Premature births comprised 8% of the material in the present investigation. The caries morbidity was greater in children who had been born prematurely, and also among children who had suffered illnesses as infants, in comparison to normal-term births and healthy children. Caries morbidity was clearly correlated with bottle-feeding and with the use of rubber pacifiers. Children who had never been bottle-fed had a caries morbidity of 15%. Children fed up to three times per day with a bottle had a morbidity of 18%, while in children bottle-fed more than three times daily the figure was 31%. Children with caries had received bottle-feeding for an average of 18 months; caries-free children for 14.2 months.

In summary, all of these results seem to indicate that natural nourishment with mother's milk aids caries resistance. However, a more exact analysis of the study material shows that the bottle-fed children in most cases had received *sweetened* bottle milk, and that they frequently were also given sugar-coated pacifiers. Naturally nourished children do not have a higher resistance to caries. Rather, bottle-fed children have a higher caries activity. 57% of the 601 children received "sweetened pacifiers" up through the fifth year of life. In the socioeconomically disadvantaged subgroup this figure was 72%! Rampant caries was twice as frequent among those children who were quieted down by means of "sweetened pacifiers" (prolonged sugar clearance).

The total avoidance of breast-feeding or the early cessation of breast-feeding *enhances* the possibility of an increase in caries activity, because the child is then more often quieted by bottled milk with sugar added, or by a sugar-coated pacifier. The administration of vitamins alone had no effect upon caries resistance. Sweetened vitamin-syrup preparations, however, did increase caries activity.

These investigations also demonstrate how important it is that young mothers receive professional advice about teeth.

Sweets also play a very significant cariogenic role in children. The following investigations[1], which were carried out in England on 4,533 middle class children aged 7 to 11 years, point up the deleterious effects of giving a child food or drinks after going to bed. Of the 4,533 children studied, the following percentages ate or drank after going to bed:

2,054 (45.3%) always
2,050 (45.2%) sometimes
  209 (9.5%) never.

These "after going to bed" snacks were classified as follows:

13.8% water only
59.8% sugar water, sweetened milk
55.9% bread, biscuits, sweets
26.5% fruits.

The caries incidence of the "always" group was significantly higher (16–21%) than that of the "never" group. Complete freedom from caries was observed twice as often among the "never" group. The oral hygiene condition was somewhat poorer in the "always" group, but there were no significant differences in gingival inflammation in the "never" group.

Sugar clearance:

> A trucker drove mile after mile,
> Consuming soft drinks all the while.
> He had long oral clearance
> And thus his appearance
> Was better if he *didn't* smile!

[1] Brit. dent. J. 130, 288; 1971.

Saliva Flow Rate

The oral fluid (OF) is a mixed secretion product derived from the three main salivary glands and the accessory (mucosal) salivary glands. The saliva may be either serous or mucous, according to its mucoid content.

Functions:

1. OF lubricates for the act of swallowing, for chewing and for phonetics.

2. OF protects the oral mucosa surfaces.

3. The OF brings soluble foodstuffs into solution; this in turn activates taste perception and also stimulates saliva flow.

4. OF minimizes dissolution of the teeth, thanks to its supersaturation with Ca^{++} and PO_4^{---}.

5. OF has a role to play in maintaining the body's water balance: the sensation of thirst is stimulated if saliva secretion is decreased.

6. OF rinses and cleans the oral cavity and shortens sugar clearance time.

7. OF enhances pre-digestion of foodstuffs through the action of its salivary enzymes.

Saliva secretion rate

One often reads that approximately 1,500 ml of oral fluid is secreted per 24-hour period. This figure is much too high. It is derived by extrapolation from the daytime flow rate, which is considerably greater than the night time flow rate.

Screenby[1] has provided the following data:

Total amount secreted during 8 hours of sleep	15 ml	= 0.03 ml/min
Total amount secreted during stimulation (eating) about two hours per day	300 ml	= 2.5 ml/min
Total amount secreted during waking hours, but without stimulation (14 hours)	400 ml	= 0.47 ml/min
	Total 700 ml	

The percentage of the total amount of oral fluid secreted by the three main salivary glands and the accessory mucosal glands varies during stimulation.

[1] Int. dent. J. 18, 812; 1968.

Flow rate of parotid saliva and non-parotid saliva (ml/min)

N = 63 adults	Parotid saliva	Oral fluid minus parotid saliva	Total
Unstimulated	0.072 (33%)	0.146	0.218
Stim. with lemon	0.756 (40%)	1.102	1.858
Stim. with sour grapes	1.515 (51%)	1.490	3.005

When the subject is at rest, OF production is approximately 0.2 ml/min. Under active stimulation, the flow of oral fluid increases about 15 times (ca. 3.0 ml/min). In a quiet subject, the parotid gland accounts for about 33% of the total production of oral fluid. On the other hand, with active stimulation, the parotid volume accounts for 51% of the total output.

During very minimal stimulation, the percentage output by the various salivary glands in a different investigation was as follows:

Submaxillary gland	41%
Sublingual gland	2%
Parotid gland	26%
Accessory mucosal glands	31%

In view of this data, one can see that in the unstimulated condition the chemical and physical characteristics of saliva produced by glands other than the parotid appear to be more important than those of parotid saliva itself.

Chemical composition of the oral fluid

Characteristically, the oral fluid exhibits a variable composition. Investigations of the make-up of the fluid have proven difficult because the organic and inorganic components vary with the degree of stimulation of the several glands. Once collected, if fresh oral fluid is then allowed to set, its mucoids depolymerize and the viscosity of the fluid is quickly lost. The very process of centrifugation employed for separating the salivary constituents can alter the OF. Alterations also occur through the action of bacterial enzymes, as a result of CO_2 loss, etc.

Water content of OF	99.4%	
Soluble components	0.5%	organic 0.3% inorganic 0.2%
Insoluble components	0.1%	(epithelial cells, leucocytes, food debris, bacteria)
Lowering of freezing point	0.3° C.	

Measurement of Saliva Flow Rate

Subject: _____

Age: _____

Examiner: _____

Date: _____

This exercise is best carried out in groups of two.

1. Determination of the pH of resting oral fluid and the flow rate of saliva, both resting and stimulated

Examiner weighs the measuring vessel. Subject sits on the treatment chair. Examiner now determines the salivary pH of the subject by placing pH indicator paper strips beneath the tongue. Next, start the stopwatch. Have the subject lean his upper body forward and allow his oral fluid to drip into the collection vessel. Subject should not move his tongue, and should not think about steak, or lemon! Depending upon the subject's flow rate, collect OF for 5 to 10 minutes. The total amount (total weight) of saliva is now determined by the examiner, according to the following formula;

weight of vessel with saliva minus weight of empty vessel = total amount of saliva.

Enter your results below.

Initial pH of resting saliva   _____

Unstimulated saliva flow rate   _____ ml/min.

(calculate from the 5–10 min value)

2. Maximum flow rate during stimulation

Now the subject's saliva flow rate is stimulated maximally by lemon juice, chewing gum etc. As soon as active, stimulated secretion has begun, the OF should be collected by having the subject clear all saliva into the collection vessel for 5 minutes. Subject need not be seated in the treatment chair during this time. No saliva should be swallowed!

Next, the examiner determines the pH of stimulated OF (stimulated saliva).

The total amount of saliva is determined by weighing the vessel after the 5-minute collection period is completed.

Maximum pH of stimulated saliva   _____

Stimulated saliva flow rate   _____ ml/min.

Instructor's signature: _____

Discussion of Results

Saliva flow rate

In 15 subjects, the resting saliva flow rate was 0.36 ± 0.21 ml/min., with an average pH of 6.8 ± 0.7.

Stimulation increased the flow rate to 3.71 ± 1.07 ml/min. The large standard deviation makes it clear that the degrees of stimulation varied greatly (0.75 to 7.3 ml/min.) Stimulated oral fluid pH was 7.4 ± 0.71. Compare these figures with those in the literature. Consult the book by Afonsky[1].

The mechanical cleansing potential, and even more the alkalinizing potential and acid-neutralizing capacity of stimulated saliva become readily apparent from these studies.

---

[1] Afonsky, D.: Saliva and its relation to oral health. A survey of the literature. University of Alabama Press, 1961.

Additional literature

Andersson, R.: The flow rate, pH and buffer effect of mixed saliva in schoolchildren. Odont. Revy 23, 421; 1972.

Periodontal Destruction–Radiographic Appearance

Instruction Sheet

XIII-1: Periodontal destruction – radiographic appearance

Exercise and Data Sheet

XIII-1: Measurement of bone loss on radiographs

Result Sheet

XIII-1: Periodontal destruction – radiographic appearance

Material

Student: clinic kit, personal radiographic survey, ruler or millimeter paper strips

Instructor: x-ray viewboxes, one radiographic survey per student from patients with periodontal disease.

Program

1. Introduction to today's topic

2. Exercises

3. Taking of impressions of selected subjects for construction of palatal plates

Periodontal Destruction-Radiographic Appearance

Quantitative radiographic assessment of the periodontium can be of significance, both epidemiologically, and in terms of judging the effectiveness of treatment performed to control periodontal disease.

Engelberger et al.[1] have provided a review of the various measurement systems. For clinical purposes, the classification according to Rateitschak[2] takes little time, although it is a relatively gross procedure. Four degrees of bone loss ar differentiated:

Grade I – radiographically detectable bone loss on one (!) root surface of a tooth, involving no more than the cervical ¼ of the root.

Grade II – bone loss involving up to half the root length

Grade III – bone loss extending over more than half the root length

Grade IV– more severe than Grade III.

All the teeth in the radiographic survey are scored. Missing teeth are assigned Grade II.

In order to assess more discrete alterations of the periodontal bone, for example the arrest of further bone loss by a periodontal treatment procedure, the method of Schai et al.[3] is useful. The authors measure the degree of bone loss in terms of root length (root length = distance from CEJ to root apex). Their data are expressed in percent and are measured with a graduated ruler.

Various x-ray projection angles change the apparent root length as well as the apparent degree of bone loss. Thus, if bone loss is measured as a percent, only small errors will exist among the various projections. Radiographic bone loss is always somewhat more pronounced than the actual osseous relationships in vivo.

Procedure

Using a ruler, the maximum bone loss is measured on a randomly selected root surface, and expressed as a percent of the total root length. One could also, of course, determine the minimal intraalveolar root length, subtract this from the total root length, and express the difference as a percentage of that total length.

[1] Engelberger, A., Rateitschak, K. H., and Marthaler, T. M.: Zur Messung des parodontalen Knochenschwundes. Helv. odont. Acta 7, 34; 1963.

[2] Rateitschak, K. H., Dossenbach, W. F. and Mühlemann, H. R.: Der Grosse Parodontosestatus. Schweiz. Mschr. Zahnheilk. 76, 621; 1966.

[3] Schai, O., Waerhaug, J., Loevdal, A. and Arno, A.: Alveolar bone loss as related to oral hygiene and age. J. Periodont. 30, 7; 1959.

The cementoenamel junction (CEJ) is an easy landmark to find on the radiograph. Interdental bone loss is measured with respect to an imaginary line connecting the CEJ and the root apex. The normal distance from the CEJ to the crest of the alveolar ridge (approx. 1 mm) can be disregarded when you calculuate the percentages.

Illustration of landmarks

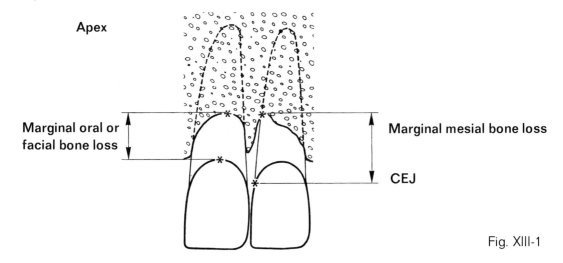

Fig. XIII-1

Crowns, post crowns and cervical restorations may render identification of the CEJ difficult. When that is the case, you should try to estimate the location of the CEJ by comparing adjacent and homologous teeth.

In studies where the goal was to determine the dependency of tooth mobility on bone loss, the intraalveolar root length was given as a percent of the total length of the tooth. This was done because tooth mobility measurements are made at the incisal region and not at the CEJ[1]. In healthy subjects, the intraalveolar root length is about 60–70% of the tooth length.

[1] Engelberger, A., Rateitschak, K. H., und Marthaler, T. M.: Zur Messung des parodontalen Knochenschwundes. Helv. odont. Acta 7, 34; 1963.

Measurement of Bone Loss on Radiographs

Subject: _____

Age: _____

Examiner: _____

Date: _____

1. On your own radiographic survey, measure the bone loss on all teeth. Measure the distance in millimeters from the proximal CEJ to the tip of the interdental alveolar septum, and subtract 1 mm from this value. Then measure the distance from the orofacial CEJ to the orofacial alveolar margin, in millimeters, and subtract 1 mm from this figure. (Normally, the distance from the CEJ to the marginal bone is 1 mm, which is why the 1 mm is subtracted.) Enter the normal bone height into the chart as "zero" (1 minus 1). Cross out any missing teeth and do not evaluate the third molars.

17   16   15   14   13   12   11   21   22   23   24   25   26   27

47   46   45   44   43   42   41   31   32   33   34   35   36   37

Radiographic bone loss:

$\overline{x}_{total}$ = bone loss on the left side (x_{1e}) _____

$\overline{x}_{total}$ = bone loss on right side (x_{rl}) _____

2. At how many places was bone loss evident?   _____

3. Can bone loss be detected radiographically where recession of the marginal gingiva is present? (compare with Exercise VI)

Distinctly detectable   [   ]

Faintly detectable   [   ]

Not detectable   [   ]

4. Radiographic survey of a patient with periodontal disease

Survey no. _____

Patient age: _____

Determine the Radiographic Index (Degree of bone loss) by estimating the bone loss Rateitschak-Mühlemann system). Missing teeth are scored as Grade II. Do not evaluate the third molars. Calculate the mean bone loss for the 28 teeth. Transform this figure into a percent of bone loss (Grade I bone loss = 25%, Grade II bone loss = 50%., etc.).

17	16	15	14	13	12	11		21	22	23	24	25	26	27
47	46	45	44	43	42	41		31	32	33	34	35	36	37

Mean bone loss $\bar{x}_{28}$ = _____

Mean bone loss in *percent* $\bar{x}$ = _____

5. Using the same radiographic survey as in question 4, determine the radiographic bone loss not by estimating, but rather by measuring on all 28 teeth. Consider missing teeth as having 50% loss. Enter your data in the chart below.

17	16	15	14	13	12	11		21	22	23	24	25	26	27
47	46	45	44	43	42	41		31	32	33	34	35	36	37

Mean bone loss in percent $\bar{x}_{28}$ = _____

Compare these percentages with those which you calculated in question 4, above. Are there differences?

Instructor's signature: _____

Periodontal Destruction–Radiographic Appearance

1. Bone loss was determined in 16 students, aged 22 to 26 years. Averages were:

$\bar{x}_{total}$ = 0.61 mm ± 0.68 mm (0.0 – 2.9)

$\bar{x}_{left}$ = 0.62 mm ± 0.62 mm (0.0 – 2.6)

$\bar{x}_{right}$ = 0.58 mm ± 0.76 mm (0.0 – 3.2)

2. In every student, bone loss was radiographically detectable in at least one area.

3. Bone loss was not detectable radiographically in regions where slight recession of the marginal gingiva was clinically evident.

4./5. The exercises using radiographic surveys from periodontal patients demonstrated the difficulties associated with attempting to measure bone loss precisely on radiographs. The CEJ landmark is often invisible.

Results from nine periodontal patients:

Estimation of degree of bone loss	32 ± 9%
Measurement of bone loss	29 ± 11%

Thus, the two procedures are equally valid. The estimation method takes less time!

The X-Ray "Eye" Sees Better:

'Super-Dentist' examined with speed,
Declaring: "For treatment, no need"!
But if time he would take
Some x-ray to make
He'd shudder when them he would read.

Occlusion

Instruction Sheets

XIV-1: Malocclusion: Definition and frequency
XIV-2: Occlusal diagnosis. Premature contacts, contacts in lateral excursion
XIV-3: Enamel abrasion and attrition
XIV-4: Malocclusion and gingivitis

Exercise and Data Sheets

XIV-1: Epidemiology of malocclusion
XIV-2: Diagnosis of premature occlusal contacts
XIV-3: Occlusal attrition facets
XIV-4: Malocclusion and gingivitis

Results Sheets

XIV-1: Discussion of results
XIV-2: Results of the occlusal diagnosis
XIV-3: Occlusal attrition facets
XIV-4: Malocclusion and gingivitis

Material

Student: clinic kit, personal plaster model with complete occlusal surfaces, ruler, compass

Instructor: colored typewriter ribbons, microscope slides

Program

1. Discussion of results from Exercise XIII, "Periodontal Destruction – radiographic appearance"

2. Introduction to today's topic

3. Exercises

4. Insertion of palatal plates by instructors. Taking of cytological smear from palatal marginal mucosa. Crevicular fluid determination on left palatal M* units. SBI determination on right palatal M units.

* refer to PMA index, Exercise VII.

Occlusion–Definitions[1]

Occlusion

Static tooth contact (bite position) without reference to the position of the mandible.

Habitual Occlusion

Tooth contact during habitual, forceful and maximal static jaw closure. Usually maximal intercuspidation in the most cranial position of the mandible. Achieved by biting hard together in the most comfortable position.

Occlusion in Centric* Relation

Tooth contact when the mandible is positioned symmetrically with respect to the cranial base, in an unforced, retruded position. (Can be routinely achieved only in patients with no history of or clinical manifestations of temporomandibular joint symptoms, e. g., pain.)

Premature Contact

A premature contact is present if occlusion in centric relation occurs only upon one or a few teeth. This is also called a premature occlucal contact.

Lateral occlusion

The occlusal contacts at a lateral position of the mandible.

Interference

Tooth contact which disturbs the smooth movement of the teeth upon each other during various mandibular excursions.

Working Side

The chewing side of the dentition. On the working side, the occlusion can be supported in several areas, e. g., there may be occlusal contact on several pairs of antagonistic teeth in the lateral position of the mandible, or there may be contact only on the cuspids (cuspid guidance).

Non-working Side

Balancing side. Lateral occlusal contacts may or may not be present.

---

[1] See also: Ramfjord, S. P., Ash, M. M.: Occlusion. W. B. Saunders Comp., London, 1966, and Physiologie und Therapie der Okklusion. Quintessenz, Berlin, 1968.

* Translator's note: In Europe, centric does not imply "at greatest intercuspidation."

Malocclusion

Definition and Frequency

Even now there is no one generally accepted definition of malocclusion (bite anomalies and tooth position anomalies). Angle[1] was the first to define the normal occlusion and variations from it. His normal occlusion is an ideal occlusion, and is one which is rarely seen in practice.

Malocclusion may be due to either bite anomalies or anomalies of tooth position.

1. Bite Anomalies

a) Disturbances in the anteroposterior relationship of the dental arches; the Angle Class II and Class III malocclusions.

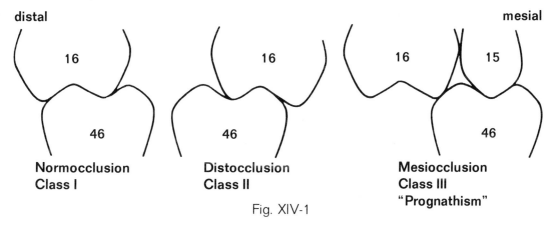

Fig. XIV-1

b) Disturbances in the transversal relationships of the dental arches in the anterior or the posterior segments (e. g., anterior cross-bite, posterior cross-bite etc.).

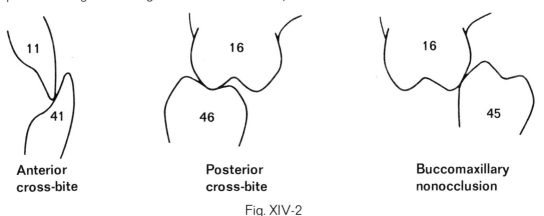

Fig. XIV-2

[1] Dent. Cosmos 41: 248–264; 350–357, 1899.

c) Disturbance in vertical relationship: anterior overbite of greater than half the crown length of the lower incisors (sometimes called "deep bite," or "closed bite." The incisal edges of the mandibular incisors may even contact the palatal soft tissue in severe cases). Overbite is often combined with a sagittal anomaly called overjet. Overjet and overbite = 0 in an ent-to-end anterior bite relationship.

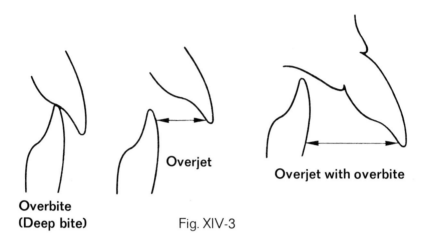

**Overbite
(Deep bite)**   Fig. XIV-3

Overjet

Overjet with overbite

An additional vertical occlusal anomaly is the open bite (see Fig. XIV-4), which may be anterior and/or posterior (infraocclusion).

2. Anomalies of Tooth Position

The tooth crown may be

   rotated (Ro)

   tipped mesially or distally (Tipping, Ti).

Anterior tooth crowns may be

   protruded to the labial   (protrusion, Pr)
   retruded   (retrusion, Re)
   incompletely erupted   (infraocclusion, IO)
   supererupted (supraocclusion, elongation, SO).

Several of the tooth position anomalies, such as crowding, cuspid prominence and malposition of cuspids and bicuspids are frequently observed. When there has been no loss of teeth, open contacts (diastema, "spacing") are more of a rarity (see Fig. XIV-4).

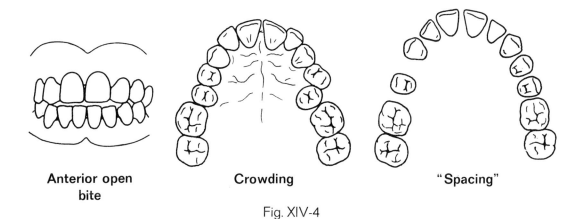

| Anterior open bite | Crowding | "Spacing" |

Fig. XIV-4

Malocclusion, in epidemiological terms, is a characteristic of the reciprocal relationship of the dental arches and the teeth. Another aspect of malocclusion, namely the relationships of the dental arches as such to fixed points on the skull has not yet been adequately studied epidemiologically.

Frequency of malocclusion

Because of the uncertainty as to what "variation from the norm," or pathology, really means, the figures available on the frequency of malocclusion show considerable variation. If we compile all the data from 16 independent studies (1921–1966) on a total of 23,500 subjects, we find a

Malocclusion frequency of 61%.

But this does not mean that all these people require treatment. According to Hotz[1], for example, only 27% of schoolchildren in Switzerland are in need of treatment, 6% because of a Class II malocclusion, 2% because of a Class III, and 19% because of crowding.

Frequency of malocclusion of the various Angle classes. Summary of the results from 14 investigations (a total of over 16,000 children and adolescents).

Anomalies within Class I	41 %	14 – 66 %
Class II	21 %	10 – 29 %
Class II ("closed bite")	4.3%	2.3 – 5.0%
Class III	3.8%	1.0 – 9.4%

[1] R. Hotz: Orthodontie in der täglichen Praxis. Hans Huber, Bern, 4th Edition, 1970.

Among 2,500 schoolchildren in the city of Zurich, Mansbach[1] found:

Normal, "good occlusion"	8.2%
Slight deviation from the norm	21.6%
Overbite (extreme overbite 3.9%)	55.5%
Anterior open bite	5.7%
Crowding (severe in 7.9%)	30.6%
Anterior cross-bite	8.9%
Class I (including cusp-to-cusp bite)	80.0%
Class II	17.2%
Class III	1.8%

Malocclusion in the primary dentition

A summary of the results from eight investigations on 6,378 children aged 2 to 6 years reveals a frequency of 29.5% (range: 17.2–66.1%).

There are no significant differences in the incidence of malocclusion whether one is studying city-dwellers, rural populations or primitive societies. Angle Class II malocclusions do appear to be less frequently encountered in American Indians and in Eskimos.

Malocclusion and fluoridation of drinking water

Five investigators found no decrease in the frequency of malocclusion in areas where fluoridated water was consumed; three investigators reported a somewhat lower prevalence[2].

The most recent epidemiological study of 1,609 Finnish children[3] gave the following results:

Frequency of malocclusion in

Primary dentition	20.1%
Mixed dentition	38.9%
Permanent dentition	58.0%

Details may be observed from the Table on the next page. By referring to the data in the latter Table, it becomes obvious that crowding, overjet and overbite are more frequent with increasing age, but the same is not true of anterior cross-bites, nor of lateral (posterior) cross-bites. Anterior open bite decreases with age.

[1] Mansbach, H.: Die Häufigkeit von Gebissanomalien bei Schulkindern. Med. Diss., Zürich 1938.

[2] Ast et al., Am. J. Orth. 48, 106; 1962.

[3] Finn. dent. J. 66, 223; 1970.

Sex differences exist only with respect to crowding in the maxilla, which is more frequent in girls.

Some work has been done with the development of occlusion indices and computer-analyzed cephalograms. These have been used only occasionally to date.

Malocclusions in primary, mixed and permanent dentitions (Finn. dent. J. 66, 223; 1970).

		primary	mixed	permanent
Class I	Crowding	1.2	9.1	16.6
	Spacing	0.6	2.6	2.4
	Anterior open bite	6.4	2.9	2.8
	Deep overbite	1.2	3.9	2.8
	Anterior cross-bite	0.6	1.7	1.3
	Transversal anomaly	3.4	5.6	7.2
	Other Class I anomalies	0.2	2.4	1.7
		13.6	28.3	34.8
Class II		4.3	6.8	17.2
Class II "closed bite"		1.6	2.4	4.8
Class III		very seldom	0.1	0.4
Not classified		0.6	1.3	0.8
	Total	20.1%	38.9%	58.0%

Malocclusion:

> The teeth leaned this way and that
> In a jaw neither skinny nor fat.
> This child from Minusio
> Had inherited protrusio
> From his mother, whose smile was worse yet!

Additional literature

The prevalence of malocclusion in Swedish schoolchildren. Scand. J. dent. Res. 81, 12–20; 1973.

Orthodontic need of treatment of Swedish schoolchildren from objective and subjective aspects. Scand. J. dent. Res. 81, 81; 1973.

Literature dealing with occlusion indices;

Salzmann, J.: Handicapping malocclusion assessment to establish treatment priority. Amer. J. Orthodont. 54, 749–765; 1968.

Grainger, R.: Interrelations of malocclusion manifestations (mathematical elucidation of malocclusion syndromes). Adv. oral Biol. 3, 145–184; 1968.

Solow, B. and Helm, S.: A method for tabulation and statistical evaluation of epidemiological malocclusion data. Acta Odont. Scand. 26, 63; 1968.

Freer, T. J. and Adkins, B. L.: New approach to malocclusion and indices. J. dent. Res. 47, 1111; 1968.

Curilović, Z.: Einfluss der experimentellen Eckzahnführung auf die Zahnbeweglichkeit. Med. Diss., Zürich 1971.

Engelberger, A., Rateitschak, K. H., Mühlemann, H. R.: Diagnostik und Therapie bei funktionellen Störungen im Kausystem. Schweiz. Mschr. Zhk. 70, 586; 1960.

Epidemiology of Malocclusion

Subject: _____

Examiner: _____

Date: _____

Frequency of tooth position anomalies

1. Enter any anomalies of tooth position into the chart. You should analyze the plaster models at home in advance! Compare your findings on the models with what you see clinically.

 – Rotation (Ro)
 – Variation in crown position: tipping (Ti), protrusion (Pr), retrusion (Re)
 – Cross-bite (Cr), or buccal nonocclusion (BN)
 – Vertical anomalies of individual teeth: supereruption (SE)

18	17	16	15	14	13	12	11		21	22	23	24	25	26	27	28
48	47	46	45	44	43	42	41		31	32	33	34	35	36	37	38

What are the occlusal relationships in the anterior region?

2. Measure the vertical overbite in the anterior region: _____ mm

   Measure the horizontal overjet in the anterior region: _____ mm

3. Frequency of bite anomalies

Determine and note the type of bite relationship:

Neutral bite: bl (bilateral)
Distal bite: ul (unlateral)
Mesial bite: ul or bl
Posterior cross-bite: ul or bl

Deep overbite   (group of teeth)
Open bite   (group of teeth)
End-to-end bite   (group of teeth)

Discussion of the Results

Findings from 43 students are, of course, not representative. The purpose of the exercise was merely to make course participants aware of the large variability in tooth position.

1. The frequencies with which the various anomalies of tooth position appeared were:

Rotation (of one or more teeth)	29 times
Tipping	30 times
Protrusion	7 times
Retrusion	6 times
Cross-bite of single teeth	3 times
Buccal nonocclusion of single teeth	4 times
End-to-end bite	0 times
Overjet	2 times

2. Occlusal relationships in the anterior region were as follows:

   The vertical overbite was 3.9 ± 2.9 mm, with a range from 1.0–11.0 mm.

   The overjet was 2.4 ± 2.1 mm; range = 0–7 mm.

3. Frequency of bite anomalies

Class I	23 times bilateral
Class II	8 times unilateral
	10 times bilateral
Class III	1 time bilateral
Posterior cross-bite	0 times
Overbite	6 times
Open bite	0
End-to-end bite	1 time

Diagnosis of Premature Occlusal Contacts (occlusion in centric relation, CR)

Subject: _____

Age: _____

Examiner: _____

Date: _____

Procedure

Examiners in groups of three will be assigned to selected patients, each of whom has a premature occlusal contact (usually, students can be found who meet this stipulation).

The three examiners should first try "teamwork" to determine which pair of antagonistic teeth contact prematurely. If all members of the examining team agree on the two teeth which are involved in the prematurity, the occlusal surface of the maxillary tooth in question should be sketched on page 227 by the best artist in the group. All anatomical details should be included, and the drawing should be at least 8 X 8 cm in dimension. The different surfaces of the tooth should be identified on the margin of the sketch.

Now, without any help or influence from the other two examiners, each examiner should sketch in with a pencil the position of the premature contact where he believes it to be. See the instructions below! It is important to have the proportions correct!

The findings of the separate examiners should then be compared. They will surely not be identical. The group should now try to come to some agreement as to the true position and shape of the premature contact, and then sketch this in its final form, using a red pencil.

Instructions for detection of premature contacts

a) Position the seated patient so that the head is leaning slightly backwards and yet at the same time is laterally symmetrical. The examiner should stand to the side and behind the patient.

b) While grasping the patient's chin laterally with both hands, guide the mandible through various movements until passive opening is achieved, i. e., until the patient can permit the examiner to open and close the mandible, in a "tap-tap-tap" procedure.

c) Using both hands, and yet with almost no pressure, move the relaxed mandible in its natural rotation movement toward the maxilla until the dental arches make their very first contact. If contact occurs on only *one* tooth, you have located a premature contact in centric relation. You may ask the patient to help you localize the premature contact, e. g., "Is it on the left, or on the right, or in the anterior region"? An experienced clinician can actually *hear* a premature contact (a double tone is evident). Very minimal prematurities can be detected through the use of an occlusal vibrator ("Equilibrator")[1].

d) Try to position the mandible so that contact is maintained upon the prematurity, without "slipping off" of it into habitual occlusion.

e) Now ask the patient to actively and completely bite the jaws together. Observe the amount and direction of mandibular shift as the patient moves from centric relation into habitual occlusion with maximum intercuspidation.

f) Try to mark the premature contact using red typewriter ribbon. Don't let the patient slip into habitual occlusion.

g) Determine the direction and estimate the size of the sliding movement into habitual occlusion, in millimeters. Enter both values on the chart.

This "Premature Contact" exercise will first be attempted on selected subjects. But how common are premature contacts in general? We will try to answer this question during the next exercise, when the students will be examining each other.

Contact in Lateral Occlusion

This investigation should be carried out with the students in groups of two. Move the mandible about 5 mm to the left, then to the right, with the teeth in contact, until the buccal surfaces of the maxillary and mandibular bicuspids form part of the circumference of the same imaginary circle (see Fig. XIV-5).

In this position, where do contacts exist on the working side? on the balancing side? (The patient's remarks will help you here.) "Is there still some air between the teeth"? "Do you feel a particular tooth with the mandible in lateral occlusion"?

Mark the lateral movements with colored ribbon (typewriter ribbon), during both right and left movements!

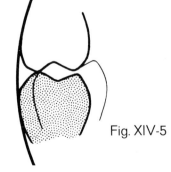

Fig. XIV-5

[1] Warwec Equilibrator. Warwec Co., P.O.Box 28, Pittsburg, Pa., U.S.A. 11662.

Occlusal Diagnosis of Premature Occlusal Contacts in Selected Subjects

Subject: _____

Age: _____

Examiner 1: _____

Examiner 2: _____

Examiner 3: _____

Date: _____

The occlusal surface of the maxillary tooth with an occlusal premature contact should be drawn in below. Include details of the occlusal anatomy; indicate mesial, distal, buccal and lingual aspects!

1. First, each examiner should sketch in the premature contact area with pencil as he (or she) sees it. Then, after discussing all of the findings, decide upon a definitive location, and sketch this in with a red pencil.

2. How long is the "slip" or glide from the premature contact into habitual occlusal position?

_____ mm

3. In which direction does this movement occur?

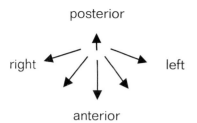

posterior

right   left

anterior

Instructor's signature: _____

Occlusal Diagnosis

Subject: _____

Age: _____

Examiner: _____

Date: _____

Students should now examine *each other,* searching for premature contacts in centric relation and in lateral position of the mandible. The lateral movement of the mandible should not exceed 5 mm.

1. Premature contacts

Did you find one? | YES | | NO |

On what teeth? _____

How long was the slide into habitual occlusal position? _____ mm

In what direction? _____

2. Contacts in lateral occlusion

On the charts below, draw lines connecting all those teeth which are in contact in lateral excursion.

a) Right side = working side

17	16	15	14	13	12	11		21	22	23	24	25	26	27
47	46	45	44	43	42	41		31	32	33	34	35	36	37

working side   balancing side

b) Left side = working side

17	16	15	14	13	12	11		21	22	23	24	25	26	27
47	46	45	44	43	42	41		31	32	33	34	35	36	37

balancing side   working side

Results of Occlusal Diagnosis

1. Premature contacts

The purpose of this investigation has been to demonstrate selected and pronounced premature contacts to the beginner, and to show how the teeth fit together. It should be pointed out that there are several distinctly different types of closed positions. There was a remarkable degree of agreement between the premature contacts diagnosed by the students and those diagnosed by the course instructors. It may thus be assumed that a considerable occlusal diagnostic sense was acquired by the students.

Of _____ students, _____ had at least one premature contact

(= _____ %).

The average slide was _____ ± _____ mm, and occurred most

often in the _____ direction.

Contacts in Lateral Occlusion

The results pertaining to occlusal contacts during lateral excursion were obtained from 34 students. Total numbers of contacts on the individual teeth are presented.

1. Right lateral position. Occlusal contact between:

No. of contacts	17	12	18	17	28	18	5		0	0	2	3	5	9	16
Tooth Number	17	16	15	14	13	12	11		21	22	23	24	25	26	27
	47	46	45	44	43	42	41		31	32	33	34	35	36	37
No. of contacts	16	11	15	18	27	17	4		0	0	3	4	3	7	15
		working side								balancing side					

2. Left lateral position. Occlusal contacts between:

No. of contacts	14	8	8	6	3	1	1		5	12	27	16	15	14	16
Tooth Number	17	16	15	14	13	12	11		21	22	23	24	25	26	27
	47	46	45	44	43	42	41		31	32	33	34	35	36	37
No. of contacts	14	6	6	6	3	1	1		3	15	25	17	14	18	16
		balancing side								working side					

The results we have just presented may be compared to those from the study by Reynolds[1]:

a) Habitual occlusion and occlusion in centric relation were the same in only 8% of randomly selected patients.

b) Habitual occlusion and occlusion in centric relation were the same in 25% of caries-free patients. In the same study, 30% had a slide of <1.0 mm; 46% >1.0 mm.

c) The fewest abrasion facets were found when habitual occlusion and occlusion in centric relation were the same.

d) In more than 50% of the cases, the mandible was supported during lateral excursion only by the cuspid teeth or by the cuspids plus the lateral incisors.

Thus, occlusions with cuspid contact only on the working side were more frequently observed than ones with posterior group function where several teeth were in contact.

e) In lateral excursion, the more quickly the bite was opened by the cuspid guidance, the fewer abrasion facets were observed. Abrasion facets were found on those opposing teeth which had premature contacts.

Occlusal Adjustment:

> The gold crown resembled a pot,
> And the bite was too high on the top.
> The dentist was thrilled.
> Through to dentin he drilled!
> But the occlusion's now right on the dot!

[1] Reynolds, J. M.: Occlusal wear facts. J. Prosth. Dent. 24, 367; 1970.

Enamel Abrasion and Attrition

Tooth hard substance is abraded physiologically during the act of chewing. This masticatory abrasion is difficult to detect. It thins the enamel covering only slightly, and, moreover, is a diffuse, even sort of wear without sharply demarcated borders. It erases the perikymata.

On the other hand, distinct, polished, sharply demarcated attrition areas are the result of friction of tooth upon tooth, or of enamel rubbing against one of the filling materials. For this reason, they are also often referred to as attrition facets or parafunctional facets.

Examples:

Proximal surface attrition facets are created as a result of the tooth mobility and the mesial wandering of the posterior teeth. Gradually, the original interdental contact *points* become abraded until they are contact *areas*, but spacing between the teeth does not occur as a result of this.

Attrition facets are more pronounced in bruxism (a parafunction).

Loss of tooth substance not due to an accident may also result from habits (e. g., seamstresses often exhibit a notch where they have continually held pins and needles between the teeth; pipe smokers will often have a neat notch to accomodate their pipe stems!). In addition, harsh abrasives and incorrect toothbrushing technique may bring about a loss of tooth substance in the form of wedge-shaped defects, primarily at the gingival margin. A combination of mechanical abrasion and chemical softening is frequently observed (erosion).

Occlusal Abrasion Facets

Subject: _____

Age: _____

Examiner: _____

Date: _____

Examine the occlusal surface complex on the plaster model and then in the oral cavity itself. Look for sharply demarcated, mirror-smooth attrition facets which have been created by parafunctional movements. Draw the attrition facets on the plaster model.

Questions

On how many teeth were distinct attrition facets evident? Where? Circle them! Cross out missing teeth.

17	16	15	14	13	12	11		21	22	23	24	25	26	27
47	46	45	44	43	42	41		31	32	33	34	35	36	37

What percent of all teeth examined had abrasion facets?   _____ %

Instructor's signature: _____

Occlusal Surface Abrasion Facets

18 students took part in this exercise. 32 ± 29% (!) of all teeth examined had clearly detectable abrasion facets on the occlusal surface. On the average, a subject had 8.6 teeth with abrasion facets.

The distribution of the abrasion facets was as follows:

Cuspids	28 times
Lateral incisors	26 times
Second bicuspids	25 times
All other teeth	19 times

Abrasion:

> There once was a baron from Altstets
> Who stuffed himself daily at banquets.
> > He grew round abdominally,
> > But inter- and approximally
> He'd created abrasion facets!

Malocclusion and Gingivitis

The relationship of malocclusion to caries, gingivitis and periodontal disease has not been subjected to adequate scientific investigation. Anomalies of tooth position may favor plaque accumulation because of the narrow embrasures they create. One has the impression that crowding of the teeth particularly enhances not only caries suspectibility but also gingivitis and a vertical type of "bone loss" within the narrow interradicular septa which are inevitably present. On the other hand, where diastemata are present, the teeth seem less prone to plaque accumulation and to the resultant caries and gingivitis.

In a study of 200 adults[1], it was shown that anomalies of tooth position create plaque-retentive areas and thus promote gingivitis. The PMA index was significantly higher where tooth positional anomalies were present.

200 patients, age 30

Anomaly of tooth position	Frequency %	Calculus Index		Plaque Index	PMA Index
		Supra-	Sub-		
not present	72.6	0.45	1.76	0.9	9.69
present	27.4	0.52	2.05	0.94	10.6
Significance P		0.1	<0.02	<0.02	<0.01

Among the three Angle classifications, there were no significant differences with respect to plaque, calculus and gingivitis.

[1] Brit. dent. J. 128, 539; 1970.

Malocclusion and Gingivitis

Subject: _____

Age: _____

Examiner: _____

Date: _____

Search for *unilateral* anomalies of tooth position, e. g., three teeth on one side of the mouth which exhibit positional abnormalities; for the sake of this discussion, we'll call these teeth x, y and z. The three homologous teeth on the opposite side of the dental arch – call them x', y' and z' – must *not* exhibit positional anomalies. Determine the degree of inflammation of the P (mesial and distal) and M (oral and facial) gingival units for all six teeth. Now compare the data for teeth x, y and z to that for x', y' and z'. (Use the Sulcus Bleeding Index for your determination of inflammation.)

Enter the SBI scores for both sides of the mouth in the charts below.

Side with anomalies of tooth position

Teeth no.

Teeth		x	y	z
P	m			
	d			
M	or			
	fac			

SBI sum for teeth x, y, z = _____

Control side (no anomalies of position)

Teeth no.

Teeth		x'	y'	z'
P	m			
	d			
M	or			
	fac			

SBI sum for teeth x', y', z' = _____

What is the difference in inflammation, in percent, on the side with the anomalies, as compared to the control side?

Instructor's signature: _____

Malocclusion and Gingivitis

17 out of 18 subjects exhibited anomalies of tooth position on one side of the dental arch, but not on the opposite side. Inflammation was more pronounced in the area of the positional anomalies in seven instances. In four cases, no difference between the anomaly side and the control side could be detected. In another seven pairs, inflammation was not apparent on either side.

In the 17 comparisons, the SBI was:

On the anomaly side:
per tooth –   1.41
per gingival unit –   0.37

On the control side:
per tooth –   0.59
per gingival unit –   0.15

Even these simple investigations demonstrate the importance of

1. anomalies of tooth position in the etiology of gingival inflammation as well as

2. the orthodontic treatment of tooth positional anomalies.

Exfoliative Cytology

Instruction Sheet

XV-1: Exfoliative cytology

Exercise and Data Sheet

XV-1: Self-investigation with the palatal plate

Results Sheet

XV-1: Discussion of the results

Material

Student: clinic kit, cement spatula

Instructor; microscope slides, cytology spatulas, fixation solution or spray, crevicular
fluid strips, ninhydrin solution

Program

1. Discussion of the results from Exercise XIV, "Occlusal Diagnosis"

2. Introduction to today's topic. Smear and fixation technique. Discussion of the palatal
   plate experiments.

3. Demonstration of subjects who have worn the palatal plate for one week. Taking of
   smears from marginal palatal mucosa. Crevicular fluid determination on palatal M
   unit of the left side; SBI determination on palatal M unit of the right side.

Exfoliative Cytology

Exfoliative cytology is employed primarily for the investigation of:

1. epithelial cells which have desquamated from a mucosal surface into a body cavity, e. g., cells within the stomach, the vagina, the oral fluid or sputum and

2. cells harvested from mucosal surfaces by various means, including scraping and pressing.

If the investigator is interested mainly in superficial epithelial alterations, the most satisfactory procedure is to use a styroflex impression, which is a pressure technique. When deeper mucosal layers must be harvested, as in the case of deeper tissue alterations, this is best accomplished by scraping with a spatula. The latter technique is employed in the study of proliferative pathological processes with a high cell turnover (e. g., dysplasia and carcinoma), and those which show dissolution of the epithelial cell layer, thus freeing single cells (e. g., bullous processes, erosive lichen planus and verrucous leukoplakia).

Practically speaking, oral exfoliative cytology aids in the early diagnosis of carcinomas. It may solidify a diagnosis of nonspecific stomatitis and vesiculo-bullous disorders. It may also confirm the presence of oral mycoses and certain precancerous alterations of the oral mucosa (e. g., lichen planus, leukoplakia, erythroplasia).

Oral exfoliative cytology has found a place in the United States as a standard diagnostic method. The Veterans Administration has a large library of pathological specimens, and provision has been made whereby once each year every active or discharged soldier may go for "mass screening," in the course of a general physical examination.

In summary, then, oral exfoliative cytology has proven to be an excellent aid in the detection, observation and differential diagnosis of inflammatory mucosal alterations, benign mucosal lesions and carcinomas.

Method

The collection of material from a suspicious lesion is performed most handily with a spatula. Fixation and staining of specimens should be carried out according to the methods of Papanicolaou[1].

Smear collection

Required armamentarium: clean microscope slides, spatula, ether-alcohol fixative solution, information sheet.
– Immediately after taking the specimen, the cellular material on the spatula must be spread without force onto a clean microscope slide.

[1] Am. J. Anat. 52, 519; 1933.

Fixation

- The slide carrying the cellular material which has been spread onto it must now be immersed in the fixative solution (ether and 96% alcohol in the ratio of 1:1). *There must not be the slightest delay* in doing this. Instead of ether-alcohol fixation, the commercially available Merckofix® Spray may be used.

- If the cellular material is allowed to dry out before fixation occurs, the specimen is then worthless because the subsequent staining procedures cannot take effect.

- Fixation should last at least 30 minutes, but should never be allowed to continue beyond 8 to 10 days. Otherwise the color reactions of the various cells diminish.

- If the specimen is to be mailed to a laboratory for diagnosis, the specimen should be removed from the fixing solution, a few drops of glycerine should be added, and a second slide or a coverslip should be applied on top of the first. The ends of the two slides can then be taped together. Pack the slide in a metal or wooden box for postal shipment.

Staining

In the staining of cell smears, clear nuclear staining and only light cytoplasmatic staining is desired. When that is the case a good visual differentiation can be made between the eosinophilic (reddish) and the cyanophilic (bluish, basophilic) components. The staining method most useful in routine oral cytology was developed by Papanicolaou. It is a technique which uses several stains. The nuclear staining substance, hematoxylin (Harris mercury hematoxylin), establishes a very good staining of the nucleus, including the nuclear fine structure. The very transparent cytoplasmic staining is obtained with orange G and an alcoholic, light green-Bismarck-eosin solution (polychrome stain). Color overlapping does not occur when this method is employed.

Results of staining according to Papanicolaou

Cell nucleus: black-brown, gray-blue to violet

Cell body: brilliant red

Cytoplasm: eosinophilic (formerly called "acidophilic") cells: pink to bright red, orange to yellowish

Cytoplasm: cyanophilic (formerly called "basophilic") cells; light blue to greenish.

Erythrocytes: brilliant red

Leukocytes: light red to light blue with dark blue nuclei

Mucous; light blue to an amorphous red

Bacteria: gray homogeneous types, or gray-blue cocci and rods.

Causes of poor staining

- Air drying before fixation
- An improper fixation solution
- A dirty slide, from which fat (oil) has not been removed
- Rinsing slcohols which are dirty and/or of improper concentration
- Stains that are too old
- Inadequate rinsing
- Drying during the staining procedure
- Staining time too long or too short
- Insufficient removal of water

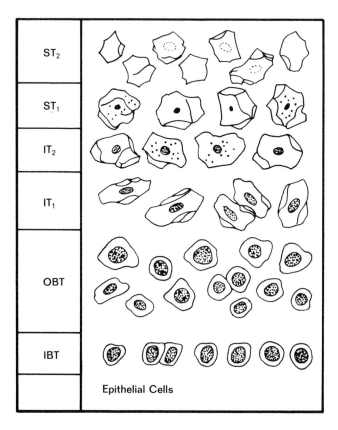

Fig. XV-1   Exfoliated oral epithelial cells. ST$_2$ No nucleus, superficial eukaryotic cells. ST$_1$ Superficial, parakeratotic cells with pyknotic nuclei. IT$_2$ Superficial cells with prepyknotic nuclei. IT$_1$ Intermediary cells. OBT Parabasal cells. IBT Basal cells.

Basal cells (cells of the "inner basal type," IBT)
They originate from the stratum basale. They are round to oval in shape, with a large, bubble-shaped, heavily staining nucleus. Their cytoplasm appears as a narrow border. The cells are cyanophilic.

Parabasal cells (cells of the "outer basal type," OBT)

These cells come from the stratum spinosum profundum. They are very similar to basal cells in shape. The cyanophilic cytoplasm is somewhat lighter. The nucleus is still quite large, and sometimes exhibits fine structuring.

Intermediary cells (cells of the "intermediate type," IT_1 and IT_2)

In this group are found the medium-sized cells of the epithelium, no longer showing the characteristics of the basal layer, but not yet exhibiting the features of superficial cells. These are oval cells, larger than the basal ones, with a tendency toward elongation (navicular cells).

The cytoplasm is usually cyanophilic. The nuclei are large and still show fine structuring (IT_1). The cells are classified as IT_2 if bubble-like nuclear alterations appear, which is a sign of beginning keratinization.

Superficial cells (cells of the "superficial type," ST)

These are the largest cells which appear in a cytological smear. They have a polygonal shape and sharply demarcated borders. The nucleus already shows the characteristics of early or total pyknosis (superficial cells with pyknotic nuclei ST_1). The cytoplasm of the immature forms is usually cyanophilic, while that of older cells is eosinophilic.

Non-nucleated particles (ST_2)

These cellular elements are the expression of a keratinization process which has already terminated. They appear as irregular, polygonal fragments, staining eosinophilic or orangeophilic. In the region of the former nucleus one frequently finds a transparent area (nuclear space).

The following general rule is valid for exfoliated cells:

The larger the nucleus of the cell, and the more cyanophilic its cytoplasm, the deeper the layer from which it originated. Of the two criteria (nuclear size and cyanophilia), nuclear size is the more important.

The Cellular Picture in Normal Oral Mucosa

Cheek and vestibule

Cyanophilic superficial (ST_1) and intermediary (IT_2) cells are present. The cell borders are folded, especially in young patients. Usually keratin particles as well as eosinophilic types of ST_1 cells are absent. The cells of the oral vestibule exhibit eosinophilia in contrast to cells of the cheek, which do not.

Hard Palate

Only orangeophilic, many-cornered keratin particles (ST_2) are present. The cells often are colonized by microorganisms.

Oral gingival epithelium (OGE)

In comparison to cheek cells, these are polyedric, small, sharply demarcated superficial cells of groups IT_2, ST_1 and ST_2. They look flattened on two sides. When the gingiva appears inflammation-free, about half of the cells in a smear will be ST_2.

Crevicular epithelium of the gingiva (sulcular epithelium)

Three cell types are present. Most dominant of all are the complexes of cyanophilic, parabasal cells (OBT), which originate from the stratum suprabasale. The OBT cells have particularly large, round nuclei. In addition, one sees cyanophilic and eosinophilic cells of the intermediary (IT_2) and superficial (ST_1) types. These originate from the oral gingival epithelium.

Dorsum of the tongue

The epithelial cells arising from the tongue, as contrasted to those from the cheek mucosa, are quite elongated. Their cytoplasm is more dense. In most cases the cells are eosinophilic. They will either have pyknotic nuclei, or no nuclei at all. Granulocytes and macrophages often accompany them. The cells are frequently covered with bacteria.

The distribution of the various cells found in cytological smear preparations from unaltered mucosa is primarily a factor of the degree of keratinization of the particular surface from which the cells came. Thus, ST_3 cells predominate in smears of the palate, but are absent in smears from the cheek. In the case of both inflammatory damage to the epithelium and neoplasia, *qualitative* cell alterations also occur.

Effects of Inflammation upon the Cells of Squamous Epithelium

Cytoplasm

– Eosinophilia occurs in the intermediary and parabasal cells (pseudo-eosinophilia).
– The cells change their normal shapes and sizes.
– Cytoplasmic vacuolization and a perinuclear halo become evident.
– Desquamation of undifferentiated epithelial cells; misshapen forms with normal nuclear structure. Cells from the lower and middle epithelial layers sometimes exhibit pseudopods. When this occurs, the cells are variously termed spider cells, tadpole cells and spindle cells.

Nucleus

Nuclear alterations in the face of inflammatory processes appear as nuclear membrane coloration, nuclear hyperchromasia, polymorphism and nuclei of various sizes. The chromatin becomes more abundant and more coarsely granulated (active nucleus). Nuclear enlargement (benign macrokaryosis), as well as multinucleation and slight deformation of the nuclear membrane also occur.

Epithelial inclusion bodies; non-epithelial elements

During inflammatory processes, epithelial inclusion elements may appear. Within a given epithelial cell, in addition to the common entrapped leukocytes, one sometimes finds several other epithelial cells. Because of their presence, the nucleus of the surrounding larger cell often is pressed against the cell membrane and assumes a sickle shape. Nonetheless, the nucleus itself does not exhibit significant alterations in size, shape (except as described in the paragraph above) or structure during inflammatory processes. There is no disturbance of the nucleus-cytoplasm ratio!

During inflammatory processes, one often observes the appearance of non-epithelial elements: polymorphonuclear granulocytes, monocytes, erythrocytes, bacterial colonies (cocci) within epithelial cells and fungi (candida albicans) which promote heterolysis (bacterial cytolysis). Leukocytes often exhibit whip-thong degeneration of their nuclei.

Literature:

Camilleri, G. E., Lange, D.: Exfoliative Cytology. A Review of its application to non-neoplastic conditions. Int. dent. J. 16, 311; 1966.

Lange, D. E., Meyer, M., Hahn, W.: Oral exfoliative cytology in the diagnosis of viral and bullous lesions. J. Periodont. 43, 433–437; 1972.

Self-Investigation with the Palatal Plate

Subject: _____

Age: _____

Examiner: _____

Date: _____

1. Findings before insertion of the palatal plate:

SB Index (M gingival unit, palatal aspect)   Crevicular fluid in millimeters (M gingival unit, palatal aspect)

17	16	15	14	13	12	11

21	22	23	24	25	26	27

2. Findings after wearing the plate for 7 days:

SB Index (M, palatal)   Crevicular fluid in mm (M, palatal)

17	16	15	14	13	12	11

21	22	23	24	25	26	27

3. Smear of marginal palatal mucosa before the experiment: date

completed [_____]

4. Smear of marginal palatal mucosa after wearing the palatal plate for 7 days   date

completed [_____]

5. This is an opportunity for you to practice making cytological smears of cells taken directly from each other. Take specimens from palatal mucosa, attached gingiva and alveolar mucosa.   date

completed [_____]

Instructor's signature: _____

Discussion of the Results

Thin palatal plates were fabricated for five of 17 students.

1. The keratinization index of the palate (percentage of non-nucleated cells) averaged 97% after the plates had been worn for 7 days. This value was practically identical to that obtained just before the plate was inserted (see also refs. 1 and 2). One may conclude from this that

a) the subjects did not wear the plates, or that

b) the plates were indeed worn, but did not injure the epithelium during the short period of wearing. The instructors in this course assume, of course, that there was student cooperation (see also point 3!).

2. According to comments by the subjects themselves, wearing of the palatal plate for one week had an insignificant effect upon the sense of taste. However, more objective criteria are needed to substantiate this.

3. Wearing of the palatal plate for one week led to irritation of the palatal marginal periodontium along the border of the plate.

The average SBI of the upper right palatal M gingival unit was 0.5 in five subjects before the experiment began. 0.75 mm of crevicular fluid was measured on the maxillary left M unit before the experiment began. After one week of wearing the palatal plate, 1.1 mm of crevicular fluid was measured, and the SBI averaged 1.1. These data point to the initiation of a slight marginal gingivitis.

Palatal Plate:

>The palatal plate was ill-fitting.
>Nowhere was it properly sitting.
>Then the question became:
>"Will the tissue be maimed"?
>To this, were no dentists admitting!

[1] Smith, P. A. E. S., James, J.: A quantitative cytophotometric study of protein-bound sulfhydryl groups in human palatal cells under experimental prosthetic conditions. Arch. oral Biol. 15, 1133; 1970.

[2] Kung, Y. S., Spranger, H.: Zytologische Untersuchungen der Alveolarmucosa unter Teilprothesen. Dtsch. zahnärztl. Z. 28, 815–818; 1973.

Tooth Mobility (TM)

Instruction Sheet

XVI-1: Tooth mobility

Exercise and Data Sheet

XVI-1: Measurement of tooth mobility

Results Sheet

XVI-1: Results of measurement of tooth mobility

Material

Student;   clinic kit

Instructor; force meter, periodontometer

Program

1. Discussion of the results from Exercise XV, "Exfoliative Cytology"

2. Introduction to today's topic

3. Exercises

Tooth Mobility

Increased tooth mobility is a cardinal sign of periodontal disease, which, by definition, leads to tooth loosening. On the other hand, it must also be stated that periodontal diseases may be even quite advanced without any evidence of increased tooth mobility! Obvious mobility in the presence of minimal bone loss leads one to suspect functional disturbances or occlusal trauma. Slight mobility in connection with severe loss of tooth supporting structure is a testimony to good biological relationships.

Increased tooth mobility is an extraordinarily sensitive early sign of alterations in the periodontal ligament whether the alterations be mechanical in nature (parafunctions) or infectious in nature (e. g., a periapical infection).

The degree of looseness of a tooth may be determined manually or with the help of the periodontometer.

Manual estimation of TM

The degree of mobility is determined using the fingernail of the index finger of both hands, or even better, with one fingernail and the end of an instrument held in the other hand. The tooth crown is moved back and forth between the two. The amount of horizontal force applied facially and orally should be slight (not more than 100–200 P.). This type of measurement is, of course, subjective. The most important thing is to compare homologous teeth!

Grade 0 = Physiological mobility
Grade 1 = Probable increase in mobility
Grade 2 = Undoubted increase in mobility
Grade 3 = Total movement ~ 0.75 mm
Grade 4 = Total movement greater than 0.75 mm; vertical mobility as well.

Periodontometry (method of Mühlemann)

A tooth which is subjected to the short-term application of various forces to both its labial and palatal surfaces, shows a biphasic movement (see Fig. XVI-1) of the crown, depending upon the force:

1. "Initial tooth mobility" (ITM)

Even with slight forces (approx. 50 to 120 P.), a relatively large horizontal total crown movement (T) results. The movement of the crown in this first phase represents the periodontal fiber system's preparation to withstand still heavier forces.

2. "Secondary tooth mobility" (STM)

Upon the application of forces greater than 100 P., the root offers greater resistance to further tipping of the tooth crown. Now the entire periodontal complex must be elastically deformed if a greater degree of crown movement is to be achieved.

On a routine basis, tooth mobility is measured only for T_{100} and T_{500}:

T_{100} = total crown movement upon application of 100 P.
T_{500} = total crown movement upon application of 500 P.

Tooth movement as dependent upon force application to the tooth crown

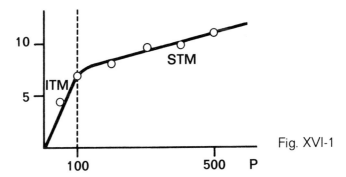

Fig. XVI-1

Normal range of physiological TM for T_{500}

(total crown movement in $\dfrac{1}{100}$ mm with 500 P. force)

Incicors	10 to 15
Cuspids	5 to 9
Bicuspids	8 to 12
Molars	4 to 8

Movements beyond these limits should be considered as pathologically increased.

Literature

Mühlemann, H. R.: Tooth mobility: a review of clinical aspects and research findings. J. Periodont. 38, 686; 1967.

Measurement of Tooth Mobility

Subject: _____

Age: _____

Examiner: _____

Date: _____

1. Using the force gauge, check out what 100–200 P actually is!

2. Attempt to see the physiological orofacial (horizontal) tooth movement of each tooth. This is not such a simple matter. Compare molars and anterior teeth. Compare homologous teeth, e. g., the two first bicuspids in the maxilla. Move the tooth crown by means of the fingernail of your left hand and an instrument in your right, or by the use of two instruments. Exert a force of about 100–200 P.

3. Determine the degree of mobility of all teeth, always comparing homologous teeth with each other.

Grade 0 Physiological mobility
Grade 1 Probably increased TM
Grade 2 Undoubtedly increased TM
Grade 3 TM to 0.75 mm
Grade 4 TM > 0.75 mm; vertical TM

Enter the TM grade above the tooth symbol in the chart below. Cross out missing teeth (X). Cross out teeth with bridges (/). Note that the chart is arranged so that you will automatically be comparing homologous teeth.

TM Grade

Maxilla	17	27	16	26	15	25		14	24	13	23	12	22	11	21
Mandible	47	37	46	36	45	35		44	34	43	33	42	32	41	31

On how many teeth was TM measured?   _____

How many teeth had Grade 1?   _____

How many teeth had Grade 2?   _____

How many homologous tooth *pairs* were
significantly different in TM?   _____

4. Estimate T_{100} on one of the periodontal patients.

Name of patient   Tooth   12 = _____
                                                          11 = _____
_____   21 = _____
                                                          22 = _____

Instructor's signature: _____

Results of Measurement of Tooth Mobility

TM was measured clinically on 314 teeth in 26 students.

18 students (70%) exhibited clinically increased tooth mobility on at least one tooth. Grade 1 mobility was found 33 times; Grade 3, four times. The causes of these increases in mobility must be clarified. All of the increases are due to alterations in the periodontium. These alterations may be inconsequential, but they may also be of a very serious nature.

Consult the radiograph! Perform functional analyses!

Remember:

a) Marginal inflammation caused by plaque does not cause increased TM.

b) Increased TM does not cause marginal inflammation.

c) Increased TM is the result of damage to the periodontium.

> *Never* say that a tooth is traumatized, or improperly loaded, or overloaded, or affected by occlusal trauma unless you can demonstrate the consequences of such traumatization, i. e., increased tooth mobility! There is no overloading without tooth mobility! "Overloading" in the absence of tooth mobility is nothing more than the fantasy of a wishful thinker!

Tooth Mobility:

I. Said Mühli of his capability
   To measure increased tooth mobility:
       "If dentists would learn
       This thing to discern,
   There'd be no more treatment futility"!

II. One dentist, not far from senility,
    Stood up and spoke out with humility:
        "Herr Doktor, I yearn
        Your art soon to learn
    But I fear my hands lack the stability"!

III. Another, with airs of gentility,
     Unimpressed by Herr Mühli's ability,
         Said with some jeers:
         "Loose molars for years
     Have never reduced my agility."

IV. Then Mühli, maintaining tranquillity,
    With a hint of sarcastic civility,
        Said: "That may be true
        But lucky for you
    That dentures do not cause sterility"!

quintessence
books

Axel Bauer/Alexander Gutowski

Gnathology

An Introduction in Theory and Practice

A new textbook, which covers all the principle chapters of the
gnathological science.
This includes: The philosophy, the functions of the stomatognatho
system, the positions and movements of the mandible, common
concepts of the ideal occlusion.
A long chapter covers the determinants of occlusion, Peter K.
Thomas wrote the chapter on the wax-up technic in organic
occlusion. In another section we have described the simulation of
jaw movements by articulators. There is a short chapter about the
Whip-Mix-Articulator and a new semiadjustable german articulator.
An in depth section is about the use of the Dentatus-Articulator
as semiadjustable instrument and a long Step-by-Step chapter
about the use of the Stuart-Computer.
The oral rehabilitation is covered by using crown and bridgework
including remount procedure. There is also a detailed description
of the oral rehabilitation by use of combined crowns and partial
prosthesis including mucostatic impressions and remount procedures. The last chapter deals with the gnathological aspects of
the full denture.

530 pages, more than 1000 illustrations (500 multi-colored).
Size: 22,5 x 25,5 cm, linen-bound with gold stamping and
protective cover, slip-case.
Price: $ 150,— plus handling and 5 % sales tax in Illinois.

quintessence
books

Milan M. Schijatschky

Life Threatening Emergencies in the Dental Practice

Review of the first German edition in the JADA 76:613, March 1968:
"Perfectly practical in his approach to the subject, the author discusses the medical aspects of treating dental patients. Since more poor risk medical patients are seen today by the dentist, the author feels that a patient's medical history should not be neglected.
The author clearly explains the importance of emergency treatment by the dentist, who can position the patient correctly, administer the right drug from a dental emergency kit, and check the patient's respiration rate and supply oxygen or institute mouth-to-mouth artificial respiration before a physician is called.
The author uses excellent illustrations to show the different situations that he discusses. The last pages of the text summarize what the dentist should do and what he should avoid. This text is a fine addition to modern dentistry. Universities might profit from it by using the material for dental education, and translations into other languages would be desirable. This is a highly impressive book that is pleasant to study and very stimulating for the student and the practitioner."
Well, here it is, the first, completely revised, English language edition. The new book has one-third more text—and twice as many illustrations—as its predecessor. The concepts discussed are absolutely up-to-date, and reflect currently held views about resuscitation, meeting the requirements of the National Conference on Cardiopulmonary Resuscitation and Emergency Cardiac Care. It's all here, in easy-to-read, easily understood form. No modern dentist should be without this book.

Foreign editions: German, Japanese
163 pp, 88 illustrations. 17×24 cm format, linen bound.
Price: $ 24.50 plus handling and 5 % sales tax in Illinois/USA.